# LOW FODMAP DIET FOOD LIST FOR BEGINNERS

A Comprehensive Guide to The Low FODMAP Diet for Beginners - From Understanding to Culinary Adventure

Christopher C. Patel

**Disclaimer Statement**

Please keep in mind that the contents of this booklet are meant for educational and recreational purposes. Every effort has been made to offer accurate, up-to-date, reliable, and thorough information. There are, however, no stated or implied assurances of any kind. Readers understand that the author is providing competent counsel. The content in this book originates from several sources. Please seek the opinion of a competent professional before using any of the tactics outlined in this book. By reading this book, the reader agrees that the author will not be held accountable for any direct or indirect damages resulting from the use of the information contained therein, including, but not limited to, errors, omissions, or inaccuracies.

# Contents

# INTRODUCTION

## Understanding the Low FODMAP Diet

*The Low FODMAP Diet is a dietary approach designed to manage symptoms of irritable bowel syndrome (IBS) and other functional gastrointestinal disorders. FODMAPs, which stands for Fermentable Oligosaccharides, Disaccharides, Monosaccharides, and Polyols, are a group of carbohydrates and sugar alcohols that can ferment in the gut, leading to symptoms such as bloating, gas, abdominal pain, and altered bowel habits.*

### What are FODMAPs?

FODMAPs encompass a variety of carbohydrates found in certain foods. This section provides an in-depth look at each category, including:

- Oligosaccharides: Fructans and Galacto-oligosaccharides
- Disaccharides: Lactose
- Monosaccharides: Fructose (in excess of glucose)
- Polyols: Sorbitol, Mannitol, Xylitol, and Isomalt

### How FODMAPs Affect the Digestive System

This section delves into the physiological processes involved when FODMAPs are consumed and reach the digestive system. Topics covered include:

- Digestion and Absorption of FODMAPs
- Fermentation and Gas Production
- Impact on Gut Motility and Sensation

*The Role of the Low FODMAP Diet*

- Understanding the Therapeutic Nature of the Diet
- Identifying Conditions that Benefit from a Low FODMAP Approach

*Research and Evidence Base*

- Overview of Clinical Studies Supporting the Efficacy of the Low FODMAP Diet
- Updates on Ongoing Research in the Field

*Who Should Consider the Low FODMAP Diet?*

- Individuals with Diagnosed IBS
- Other Gastrointestinal Conditions Suitable for the Low FODMAP Diet
- Considerations for Pregnant and Breastfeeding Individuals

*Potential Benefits and Limitations*

- Positive Outcomes in Symptom Management
- Challenges and Considerations for Long-Term Adherence

# Who Can Benefit from a Low FODMAP Diet?

*The Low FODMAP Diet is a specialized dietary approach that has demonstrated significant efficacy in managing symptoms associated with irritable bowel syndrome (IBS) and other functional gastrointestinal disorders. While individual responses to the diet may vary, several groups of individuals can particularly benefit from adopting a Low FODMAP approach.*

***Individuals with Diagnosed Irritable Bowel Syndrome (IBS):***

- ***Symptom Management:*** The primary impetus behind the Low FODMAP Diet is its effectiveness in alleviating the often-debilitating symptoms of IBS, such as abdominal pain, bloating, gas, and irregular bowel movements.

- ***Enhancing Quality of Life:*** For individuals diagnosed with IBS, implementing a Low FODMAP Diet can lead to a substantial improvement in their overall quality of life by mitigating the impact of gastrointestinal symptoms.

***Those with Functional Gastrointestinal Disorders:***

- ***Similar Symptomatology:*** Individuals with functional gastrointestinal disorders sharing symptoms akin to IBS, such as functional bloating or functional diarrhea, may find relief through the targeted elimination of high FODMAP foods.

- *Tailored Approach:* The diet offers a tailored, evidence-based approach for managing symptoms that may not respond optimally to general dietary advice.

*Individuals with Non-Responsive Gastrointestinal Symptoms:*

- *Unexplained Gastrointestinal Distress*: For those experiencing persistent gastrointestinal symptoms without a clear diagnosis, the Low FODMAP Diet can serve as a diagnostic tool to identify specific food triggers.

- *Assisting Healthcare Professionals:* This approach aids healthcare professionals in refining their diagnostic process and developing personalized dietary strategies for their patients.

*Athletes and Individuals with Specific Dietary Goals:*

- *Optimizing Performance:* Athletes, especially those sensitive to gastrointestinal discomfort during training, may find the Low FODMAP Diet beneficial in optimizing nutrition without compromising performance.

- **Achieving Dietary Goals:** Individuals with specific dietary goals, such as weight management or muscle building, can adapt the principles of the Low FODMAP Diet to meet their nutritional needs while minimizing digestive discomfort.

**Pregnant and Breastfeeding Individuals with Gastrointestinal Sensitivities:**

- **Careful Adaptation:** Pregnant and breastfeeding individuals, under the guidance of healthcare professionals, can adapt the Low FODMAP Diet to manage gastrointestinal symptoms while ensuring adequate nutrient intake for both themselves and their child.

- **Consulting Healthcare Providers:** It is crucial for pregnant or breastfeeding individuals to consult with healthcare providers before making significant dietary changes.

# CHAPTER ONE

## Definition of FODMAPs

*FODMAPs, an acronym for Fermentable Oligosaccharides, Disaccharides, Monosaccharides, and Polyols, represent a group of short-chain carbohydrates and sugar alcohols that are naturally present in various foods. These compounds are notorious for their ferment ability in the gut, a process that can lead to the onset or exacerbation of gastrointestinal symptoms in susceptible individuals.*

***Fermentable Oligosaccharides (Fructans and Galacto-oligosaccharides):***

- ***Fructans:*** Found in a variety of foods, including wheat, rye, onions, and garlic, Fructans are chains of fructose molecules linked together. Their resistance to digestion in the small intestine allows them to reach the colon, where fermentation occurs.

- ***Galacto-oligosaccharides (GOS):*** Present in legumes and certain vegetables, GOS consist of short chains of galactose molecules. They, too, reach the colon intact and undergo fermentation by gut bacteria.

### Disaccharides (Lactose):

- **Lactose:** A disaccharide sugar naturally present in dairy products, lactose requires the enzyme lactase for proper digestion. Individuals with lactose intolerance lack sufficient lactase, leading to undigested lactose reaching the colon and causing symptoms.

### Monosaccharides (Fructose in excess of Glucose):

- **Fructose:** A natural sugar found in fruits, honey, and some vegetables, fructose is typically absorbed in the small intestine. However, when present in excess of glucose, unabsorbed fructose can contribute to symptoms in individuals with fructose malabsorption.

### Polyols (Sorbitol, Mannitol, Xylitol, and Isomalt):

- **Sorbitol and Mannitol:** These sugar alcohols occur naturally in certain fruits and vegetables and are also used as sweeteners in sugar-free products. They are poorly absorbed and can lead to osmotic effects and fermentation in the colon.

- **Xylitol and Isomalt:** Additional sugar alcohols found in some fruits and sugar-free products, these compounds share the characteristic of limited absorption, contributing to their FODMAP classification.

***Significance of FODMAPs in Gastrointestinal Health:***

- FODMAPs play a pivotal role in the context of gastrointestinal health, particularly in individuals with conditions such as irritable bowel syndrome (IBS). Their resistance to absorption in the small intestine and subsequent fermentation in the colon can result in the production of gas and other byproducts, contributing to symptoms like bloating, abdominal pain, and altered bowel habits.

# Common Types of FODMAPs

*FODMAPs, or Fermentable Oligosaccharides, Disaccharides, Monosaccharides, and Polyols, encompass a range of carbohydrates and sugar alcohols that can trigger gastrointestinal symptoms in susceptible individuals. A nuanced understanding of the common types of FODMAPs is crucial for those navigating the Low FODMAP Diet and seeking relief from conditions such as irritable bowel syndrome (IBS).*

**Oligosaccharides:**

- ***Fructans:*** Found abundantly in various grains and vegetables, Fructans consist of chains of fructose molecules. Wheat, rye, onions, and garlic are notable sources. Their resistance to digestion in the small intestine contributes to their FODMAP classification.

- *Galacto-oligosaccharides(GOS):* Present in legumes, lentils, and certain nuts, GOS are short chains of galactose molecules. These compounds are known for their ferment ability in the colon, leading to gas production and other symptoms in susceptible individuals.

## Disaccharides:

- *Lactose:* Lactose, a disaccharide sugar, is primarily found in dairy products. The enzyme lactase is necessary for its proper digestion. Lactose intolerance, a common condition, arises when there is insufficient lactase to break down lactose, resulting in its fermentation in the colon.

## Monosaccharides:

- *Fructose in excess of Glucose:* While fructose is a natural sugar present in fruits, honey, and some vegetables, its malabsorption can occur when there is an excess of fructose in comparison to glucose. This imbalance can lead to symptoms in individuals with fructose malabsorption.

**Polyols:**

- ***Sorbitol and Mannitol:*** Naturally occurring in some fruits and vegetables, sorbitol and mannitol are sugar alcohols that resist absorption in the small intestine. Their osmotic effects and fermentation in the colon contribute to symptoms such as bloating and abdominal discomfort.

- ***Xylitol and Isomalt:*** Found in certain fruits and used as sugar substitutes, xylitol and Isomalt are additional sugar alcohols with limited absorption. Their classification as FODMAPs stems from their potential to ferment in the colon, impacting individuals sensitive to these compounds.

## How FODMAPs Affect the Digestive System

*Understanding the impact of FODMAPs (Fermentable Oligosaccharides, Disaccharides, Monosaccharides, and Polyols) on the digestive system is essential for individuals navigating conditions such as irritable bowel syndrome (IBS) and seeking relief through the Low FODMAP Diet. The intricate processes involved highlight the connection between FODMAP consumption and the onset of gastrointestinal symptoms.*

**Digestion and Absorption of FODMAPs:**

- *Digestive Enzyme Insufficiencies:* The journey of FODMAPs begins in the small intestine, where they encounter digestive enzymes responsible for breaking them down into absorbable components. Insufficiencies or deficiencies in these enzymes, such as lactase for lactose digestion, can result in the malabsorption of specific FODMAPs.

- *Resistance to Digestion:* Certain FODMAPs, particularly oligosaccharides like Fructans and GOS, resist complete digestion in the small intestine. This resistance allows them to reach the colon intact, setting the stage for subsequent fermentation.

**Fermentation and Gas Production:**

- *Colon Microbiota:* Upon reaching the colon, undigested FODMAPs become substrates for fermentation by the gut microbiota. This microbial activity produces gases, including carbon dioxide, methane, and hydrogen.

- *Osmotic Effects:* The fermentation of FODMAPs also results in the production of short-chain fatty acids and other byproducts, contributing to osmotic effects. This draws water into the colon, leading to increased bowel water content and potential symptoms such as bloating and diarrhea.

**Impact on Gut Motility and Sensation:**

- **Distension of the Colon:** Gas production and osmotic effects can contribute to the distension of the colon, leading to sensations of bloating and abdominal discomfort.

- **Altered Gut Motility:** FODMAPs can influence gut motility, affecting the rhythmic contractions of the intestines. This altered motility may contribute to symptoms such as abdominal pain and changes in bowel habits.

**Individual Variability in FODMAP Sensitivity:**

- **Threshold Effect:** The impact of FODMAPs on the digestive system exhibits individual variability. Some individuals may have a lower threshold for experiencing symptoms, while others may tolerate higher amounts without adverse effects.

- **Interaction with Other Factors:** FODMAP sensitivity can be influenced by factors such as stress, psychological well-being, and the overall composition of the gut microbiota.

# CHAPTER TWO

# GETTING STARTED WITH THE LOW FODMAP DIET

## Preparing Mentally and Physically for the Low FODMAP Diet

*Embarking on the Low FODMAP Diet requires more than just adjusting your food choices; it necessitates a holistic approach that encompasses mental and physical preparation. Preparing oneself mentally and physically is crucial for a successful and sustainable journey through the intricacies of this dietary strategy.*

**Understanding the Purpose and Commitment:**

- *Mental Aspect:* Begin by understanding the purpose of the Low FODMAP Diet. Recognize that it is not just about restriction but a systematic process to identify and manage triggers for gastrointestinal symptoms.

- *Physical Aspect:* Acknowledge that this dietary approach requires commitment and consistency. Clear communication with healthcare professionals and dietitians can provide a roadmap for the journey ahead.

**Educating Yourself:**

- *Mental Aspect:* Equip yourself with knowledge about FODMAPs, their sources, and their potential effects on the digestive system. This knowledge empowers you to make informed decisions and fosters a sense of control.
- *Physical Aspect:* Create a comprehensive list of high and low FODMAP foods. Familiarize yourself with food labels and ingredient lists to make informed choices while grocery shopping.

**Clearing Your Environment:**

- *Mental Aspect:* Prepare mentally by decluttering your surroundings of potential stressors. This may involve creating a supportive and understanding environment at home and work to alleviate unnecessary pressures.
- *Physical Aspect:* Physically clear your pantry and refrigerator of high FODMAP foods. This not only helps you avoid accidental consumption but also reinforces your commitment to the dietary plan.

**Planning Meals and Snacks:**

- *Mental Aspect:* Develop a positive mindset towards meal planning. View it as an opportunity to explore new recipes and discover delicious low FODMAP alternatives.

- *Physical Aspect:* Create weekly meal plans and shopping lists. Having a well-thought-out plan makes it easier to stick to the diet and reduces the likelihood of feeling overwhelmed when deciding what to eat.

**Seeking Emotional Support:**

- *Mental Aspect:* Recognize that emotions play a role in dietary success. Seeking emotional support from friends, family, or support groups can provide encouragement during challenging moments.

- *Physical Aspect:* Engage in activities that promote mental well-being, such as regular exercise, mindfulness practices, or hobbies. Physical and mental well-being are interconnected aspects of overall health.

**Establishing Realistic Expectations:**

- *Mental Aspect:* Set realistic expectations for yourself. Understand that the journey may have its ups and downs, and adjustments may be necessary along the way.

- *Physical Aspect:* Pay attention to physical signals from your body. Be patient and allow time for your digestive system to adapt to the changes.

# Consulting with a Healthcare Professional

*Embarking on the Low FODMAP Diet is a significant step towards managing gastrointestinal symptoms, but the journey is most effective when guided by the expertise of a healthcare professional. Consulting with a qualified professional is a pivotal aspect of ensuring a safe, personalized, and successful experience with the Low FODMAP Diet.*

**Establishing a Baseline:**

- *Professional Expertise:* Healthcare professionals, such as gastroenterologists, dietitians, or nutritionists, bring specialized knowledge to the table. They can assess your overall health, understand your medical history, and identify any underlying conditions that may impact your response to the diet.

- *Individualized Approach:* Your healthcare provider can tailor recommendations based on your unique health profile, taking into consideration factors such as age, existing medical conditions, and medications.

**Confirming the Diagnosis:**

- *Ruling Out Other Conditions:* Gastrointestinal symptoms may be indicative of various conditions.

A healthcare professional can perform necessary tests to rule out other potential causes, ensuring that the symptoms are appropriately attributed to conditions like irritable bowel syndrome (IBS).

- *Accurate Diagnosis:* An accurate diagnosis lays the foundation for an effective management plan. This may involve differentiating between IBS and inflammatory bowel diseases or other gastrointestinal disorders.

**Guidance on Dietary Adjustments:**

- *Interpreting Individual Needs:* Healthcare professionals can interpret the nuances of your dietary needs. They can guide you on the specifics of the Low FODMAP Diet, ensuring that it aligns with your nutritional requirements and personal preferences.

- *Avoiding Nutritional Deficiencies:* Professionals can help you avoid potential nutritional deficiencies by recommending suitable substitutes for high FODMAP foods. This ensures that the diet remains balanced and meets your nutritional needs.

**Monitoring Progress and Adjustments:**

- *Regular Follow-ups:* Periodic check-ins with healthcare professionals allow for ongoing monitoring of your progress. They can assess the effectiveness of the diet, make necessary adjustments, and address any emerging concerns.
- *Addressing Challenges:* If challenges arise during the implementation of the Low FODMAP Diet, healthcare professionals can provide practical solutions, ensuring that the dietary plan remains manageable and sustainable.

**Psychological Support:**

- *Addressing Emotional Well-being:* Gastrointestinal conditions can have psychological implications. Healthcare professionals can offer support and resources to address the emotional aspects of dietary changes, promoting overall well-being.
- *Providing Resources:* Professionals may recommend additional resources such as support groups or mental health services to complement the dietary intervention.

# Understanding Food Labels

*One of the fundamental aspects of successfully adhering to the Low FODMAP Diet is the ability to decipher and understand food labels. As this dietary approach involves meticulous attention to the FODMAP content of various products, mastering the art of reading food labels becomes an indispensable skill. Here's a professional discourse on the importance and nuances of understanding food labels within the context of the Low FODMAP Diet.*

**Grasping the FODMAP Terminology:**

- ***Recognition of High FODMAP Ingredients:*** Individuals on the Low FODMAP Diet must familiarize themselves with common high FODMAP ingredients. Recognizing terms such as fructose, Fructans, Galacto-oligosaccharides (GOS), lactose, and polyols on food labels is pivotal.

- ***Ingredient Variations:*** Be aware of variations in ingredient names. For example, Fructans may appear as inulin or chicory root extract. Understanding these variations enhances the ability to spot potential FODMAP sources.

**Analyzing Serving Sizes:**

- **Portion Control Considerations:** Paying attention to serving sizes on food labels is crucial. Certain products may be low FODMAP in small quantities but become high FODMAP when consumed in larger amounts. This awareness aids in managing FODMAP intake effectively.

- **Adjusting Portion Sizes:** Understanding serving sizes also allows individuals to adjust their portion sizes according to their tolerance levels, promoting flexibility in food choices.

**Identifying Hidden FODMAPs:**

- **Recognition of Hidden Ingredients:** Manufacturers may use high FODMAP ingredients in unexpected products. Understanding food labels helps in identifying hidden sources of FODMAPs, contributing to a more accurate dietary strategy.

- **Processed Foods and Additives:** Processed foods may contain FODMAP-rich additives. Learning to recognize these additives on labels enables individuals to make informed decisions about the suitability of such products.

**Utilizing Certification Symbols:**

29

- *Gluten-Free and Low FODMAP Certifications:* Some products may bear certifications such as "gluten-free" or "low FODMAP." Understanding the reliability of these symbols aids individuals in making quicker and more confident choices during grocery shopping.

- *Cross-Contamination Considerations:* Recognizing potential risks of cross-contamination is crucial. While a product may be low FODMAP, shared equipment or facilities may introduce cross-contamination. Understanding labeling practices and symbols helps mitigate these risks.

**Staying Informed About Labeling Regulations:**

- *Local and International Standards:* Food labeling regulations vary across regions. Being aware of local and international standards ensures individuals can navigate labels accurately, especially when exploring products from different markets.

- *Updates and Revisions:* Labeling regulations may undergo updates or revisions. Staying informed about these changes helps individuals adapt their understanding of food labels to ensure compliance with the latest information.

# CHAPTER THREE
# FOODS TO AVOID

## High FODMAP Fruits

- *Apples:* High in fructose and sorbitol, apples are considered high FODMAP.

- *Pears:* Similar to apples, pears contain elevated levels of fructose and sorbitol.

- *Watermelon:* With both high fructose content and a high fructose-to-glucose ratio, watermelon is classified as high FODMAP.

- *Mangoes:* Rich in both fructose and sorbitol, mangoes should be avoided on a Low FODMAP Diet.

- *Cherries:* Cherries contain excess fructose, making them a high FODMAP fruit.

- *Peaches:* High in excess fructose and sorbitol, peaches are considered FODMAP-rich.

- *Plums:* Plums have elevated levels of both fructose and sorbitol, making them unsuitable for a Low FODMAP Diet.

- **Nectarines:** Similar to peaches, nectarines are high in excess fructose and sorbitol.

- **Apricots:** Dried apricots, in particular, are concentrated in fructose and sorbitol and should be avoided.

- **Mango Juice:** As a concentrated form of mango, mango juice is high in FODMAPs.

- **Pear Juice:** Like whole pears, pear juice is high in excess fructose and sorbitol.

- **Apple Juice:** With concentrated fructose, apple juice is not suitable for a Low FODMAP Diet.

## High FODMAP Vegetables

- **Onions:** Onions, including all varieties such as red, white, yellow, and shallots, are high in Fructans.

- **Garlic:** Garlic is a significant source of Fructans, contributing to its high FODMAP content.

- **Leeks:** Leeks, often used in soups and stews, contain high levels of Fructans and should be avoided.

- **Spring Onions (Scallions):** Both the green and white parts of spring onions are high in Fructans.

- **Shallots:** Similar to onions, shallots are rich in Fructans and should be excluded from a Low FODMAP Diet.

- **Artichokes:** Both globe and Jerusalem artichokes are high in Fructans, making them unsuitable for the Low FODMAP Diet.

- **Asparagus:** Asparagus contains moderate levels of Fructans, and its consumption should be limited.

- **Sugar Snap Peas:** Sugar snap peas are high in both fructose and Fructans.

- **Snow Peas:** Similar to sugar snap peas, snow peas are high in fructose and Fructans.

- **Cauliflower:** Cauliflower contains polyols, specifically mannitol, making it a high FODMAP vegetable.

- **Mushrooms:** Certain mushrooms, such as shiitake and button mushrooms, are high in polyols.

- **Brussels Sprouts:** Brussels sprouts contain moderate levels of Fructans and should be restricted on the Low FODMAP Diet.

## High FODMAP Proteins

*Proteins, in their natural state, do not contain FODMAPs. However, certain protein-rich foods may be prepared or processed with high FODMAP ingredients or cooking methods. Here's a list of protein-rich foods to be cautious about and potentially avoid due to added FODMAPs:*

- **Processed Meats:** Some processed meats may contain high FODMAP ingredients, such as garlic or onion powder, as flavor enhancers. Examples include sausages, hot dogs, and deli meats.

- **Breaded or Coated Proteins:** When proteins are coated or breaded, the coating often contains wheat or other high FODMAP flours. This includes items like breaded chicken or fish.

- **Marinated Proteins:** Proteins marinated in high FODMAP ingredients like garlic or onion may contribute to FODMAP content. Be cautious with pre-marinated meats or those prepared with high FODMAP sauces.

- **Canned Proteins:** Some canned proteins, like tuna or salmon, may have added ingredients that are high in FODMAPs. It's important to check labels for added Fructans, garlic, or onion.

- **Vegetarian Meat Alternatives:** Certain vegetarian meat substitutes, such as those made from legumes or mushrooms, can be high in FODMAPs. Check labels for ingredients that may contribute to FODMAP content.

- **Prepared or Processed Protein Snacks:** Protein bars, shakes, or snacks can contain high FODMAP ingredients such as certain sweeteners or additives. Always check labels for FODMAP content.

## High FODMAP Grains

*Grains can be a significant source of FODMAPs, particularly certain types that are high in Fructans or other fermentable carbohydrates. Here's a list of high FODMAP grains that individuals following the Low FODMAP Diet may need to limit or avoid:*

- **Wheat:** Wheat and wheat-containing products are high in Fructans. This includes items such as wheat bread, pasta, couscous, and wheat-based cereals.
- **Rye:** Rye contains Fructans and is considered high FODMAP. Rye bread and other products made with rye flour should be avoided.
- **Barley:** Barley contains Fructans and is high in FODMAPs. This includes barley-based products like certain cereals and malted products.
- **Spelt:** Spelt is a type of wheat and is high in Fructans. Products made with spelt flour, such as spelt bread, should be avoided.
- **Semolina:** Semolina, commonly used in pasta and couscous, is high in Fructans and is a high FODMAP grain.
- **Farro:** Farro contains Fructans and is considered high FODMAP. It is often used in salads, soups, or as a side dish.
- **Kamut:** Kamut is another type of wheat and is high in Fructans. Products made with kamut flour should be avoided.

- **Amarnath:** Amarnath is a pseudo cereal high in Fructans. It's often found in some gluten-free products.

- **Bulgur:** Bulgur is a form of wheat that contains Fructans and is considered high FODMAP.

- **Couscous:** Traditional couscous is made from wheat and is high in Fructans. Gluten-free alternatives, like rice or corn couscous, are suitable on the Low FODMAP Diet.

## Quinoa Breakfast Bowl

*Ingredients:*

- 1 cup cooked quinoa
- 1/2 cup lactose-free yogurt
- 1/2 cup strawberries, sliced
- 1 tablespoon chia seeds
- 1 tablespoon maple syrup

*Preparation Time:* 5 minutes

*Cooking Time:* 15 minutes (for quinoa)

*Serving Time:* 10 minutes

*Nutritional Info:* (per serving)

- Calories: 300
- Protein: 10g
- Fiber: 5g

*Instructions:*

- Cook quinoa according to package instructions.
- In a bowl, combine cooked quinoa, lactose-free yogurt, sliced strawberries, chia seeds, and maple syrup.
- Mix well and serve.

*Serving Methods:*

1. Serve warm for a cozy breakfast.
2. Make it ahead for a quick grab-and-go option.

## Low FODMAP Veggie Omelette

*Ingredients:*

- 2 large eggs
- 1/4 cup red bell pepper, diced
- 1/4 cup zucchini, grated
- 1 tablespoon chives, chopped
- Salt and pepper to taste

*Preparation Time:* 7 minutes

*Cooking Time:* 5 minutes

*Serving Time:* 12 minutes

*Nutritional Info:* (per serving)

- Calories: 180
- Protein: 12g
- Fat: 12g

*Instructions:*

- In a bowl, whisk eggs and season with salt and pepper.
- Heat a non-stick pan over medium heat.
- Add diced red bell pepper and grated zucchini to the pan. Cook for 2-3 minutes.

- Pour whisked eggs over the veggies and sprinkle with chives.
- Cook until the edges set, then fold the omelette in half.
- Serve hot.

**Serving Methods:**

1. Top with a dollop of lactose-free sour cream.
2. Wrap the omelette in a gluten-free tortilla for a portable option.

# Blueberry Almond Smoothie

**Ingredients:**

- 1/2 cup blueberries
- 1 tablespoon almond butter
- 1 cup lactose-free milk
- 1/2 banana (under-ripe), sliced
- Ice cubes

**Preparation Time:** 5 minutes

**Serving Time:** Immediate

**Nutritional Info:** (per serving)

- Calories: 250
- Protein: 8g
- Fiber: 4g

**Instructions:**

- In a blender, combine blueberries, almond butter, lactose-free milk, sliced banana, and ice cubes.
- Blend until smooth.
- Pour into a glass and serve.

*Serving Methods:*
1. Garnish with a sprinkle of chia seeds.
2. Pour into a portable cup for an on-the-go breakfast.

## Spinach and Tomato Frittata Muffins

*Ingredients:*
- 4 large eggs
- 1/2 cup spinach, chopped
- 1/4 cup cherry tomatoes, halved
- 1 tablespoon olive oil
- Salt and pepper to taste

*Preparation Time:* 10 minutes

**Cooking Time:** 15 minutes

*Serving Time:* 12 minutes

*Nutritional Info:* (per serving)
- Calories: 180
- Protein: 10g
- Fat: 12g

*Instructions:*

- Preheat the oven to 350°F (180°C).
- In a bowl, whisk eggs and season with salt and pepper.
- Heat olive oil in a pan, add spinach and cherry tomatoes, and cook until wilted.
- Grease a muffin tin and distribute the vegetable mixture evenly.
- Pour the whisked eggs over the vegetables.
- Bake for 15 minutes or until the frittata is set.
- Allow to cool slightly before serving.

*Serving Methods:*

1. Top with lactose-free shredded cheese for added flavor.
2. Serve with a side of sliced cucumber and a drizzle of balsamic glaze.

# Peanut Butter Banana Rice Cakes

*Ingredients:*

- 2 rice cakes (gluten-free)
- 2 tablespoons peanut butter (no added high FODMAP ingredients)
- 1 banana (under-ripe), sliced
- Cinnamon for sprinkling

*Preparation Time:* 5 minutes

*Serving Time:* Immediate

*Nutritional Info:* (per serving)

- Calories: 280
- Protein: 7g
- Fiber: 4g

*Instructions:*

- Spread peanut butter evenly on rice cakes.
- Top with sliced bananas and sprinkle with cinnamon.
- Enjoy as an open-faced sandwich.

*Serving Methods:*

1. Drizzle with a touch of maple syrup for added sweetness.
2. Pack in a container for a convenient on-the-go breakfast.

## Chia Seed Pudding with Berries

*Ingredients:*

- 2 tablespoons chia seeds
- 1 cup lactose-free milk
- 1/2 cup mixed berries (e.g., strawberries, blueberries)
- 1 tablespoon maple syrup

*Preparation Time:* 5 minutes (plus chilling time)

***Serving Time:*** 2 hours

***Nutritional Info:*** (per serving)

- Calories: 220
- Protein: 7g
- Fiber: 8g

***Instructions:***

- In a bowl, mix chia seeds, lactose-free milk, and maple syrup.
- Refrigerate for at least 2 hours or overnight until it thickens.
- Before serving, top with mixed berries.

***Serving Methods:***

1. Layer with lactose-free yogurt for a parfait.
2. Garnish with a sprinkle of chopped nuts for added crunch.

## Lactose-Free Greek Yogurt Parfait

***Ingredients:***

- 1 cup lactose-free Greek yogurt
- 1/2 cup granola (low FODMAP)
- 1/4 cup kiwi, diced
- 1 tablespoon maple syrup

***Preparation Time:*** 5 minutes

***Serving Time:*** Immediate

*Nutritional Info:* (per serving)

- Calories: 280
- Protein: 15g
- Fiber: 4g

*Instructions:*

- In a glass or bowl, layer lactose-free Greek yogurt with granola.
- Add diced kiwi on top.
- Drizzle with maple syrup for sweetness.
- Repeat the layers and serve.

*Serving Methods:*

1. Garnish with a few fresh mint leaves for a burst of flavor.
2. Prepare in a mason jar for a visually appealing and portable breakfast.

## Oatmeal with Banana and Cinnamon

*Ingredients:*

- 1/2 cup oats (gluten-free)
- 1 cup lactose-free milk
- 1 banana (under-ripe), sliced
- 1/2 teaspoon cinnamon
- 1 tablespoon maple syrup

*Preparation Time:* 5 minutes

***Cooking Time:*** 5 minutes

***Serving Time:*** Immediate

***Nutritional Info:*** (per serving)

- Calories: 280
- Protein: 8g
- Fiber: 5g

***Instructions:***

- Cook oats with lactose-free milk according to package instructions.
- Top with sliced bananas, cinnamon, and a drizzle of maple syrup.
- Stir well and enjoy warm.

***Serving Methods:***

1. Sprinkle with chopped nuts or seeds for added texture.
2. Serve in a hollowed-out half of a papaya for a creative presentation.

## Smoked Salmon and Avocado Toast

***Ingredients:***

- 2 slices gluten-free bread
- 2 ounces smoked salmon
- 1/2 avocado, sliced
- Chives for garnish

- Lemon wedge

*Preparation Time:* 7 minutes

*Serving Time:* Immediate

*Nutritional Info:* (per serving)

- Calories: 300
- Protein: 15g
- Healthy Fats: 15g

*Instructions:*

- Toast gluten-free bread slices.
- Top each slice with smoked salmon and sliced avocado.
- Garnish with chives and squeeze fresh lemon juice on top.

*Serving Methods:*

1. Add a poached egg on top for extra protein.
2. Serve with a side of lactose-free cream cheese for added creaminess.

# Pumpkin Spice Smoothie Bowl

*Ingredients:*

- 1/2 cup canned pumpkin (unsweetened)
- 1/2 banana (under-ripe), sliced
- 1/2 cup lactose-free yogurt
- 1/4 teaspoon pumpkin spice

- 1 tablespoon sunflower seeds (for topping)

*Preparation Time:* 5 minutes

*Serving Time:* Immediate

*Nutritional Info:* (per serving)

- Calories: 220
- Protein: 6g
- Fiber: 6g

*Instructions:*

- In a blender, combine canned pumpkin, sliced banana, lactose-free yogurt, and pumpkin spice.
- Blend until smooth.
- Pour into a bowl and top with sunflower seeds.

*Serving Methods:*

1. Add a sprinkle of gluten-free granola for crunch.
2. Drizzle with a touch of maple syrup for sweetness.

# Low FODMAP Breakfast Burrito

*Ingredients:*

- 2 gluten-free tortillas
- 2 large eggs, scrambled
- 1/2 cup spinach, chopped
- 1/4 cup lactose-free shredded cheese
- Salt and pepper to taste

*Preparation Time:* 7 minutes

*Cooking Time:* 5 minutes

*Serving Time:* Immediate

*Nutritional Info:* (per serving)

- Calories: 280
- Protein: 14g
- Healthy Fats: 10g

*Instructions:*

- Heat the tortillas in a skillet or microwave until warm.
- In a separate pan, scramble the eggs until cooked.
- Add chopped spinach to the pan and cook until wilted.
- Divide the scrambled eggs and spinach mixture between the warm tortillas.
- Sprinkle lactose-free shredded cheese on top.
- Season with salt and pepper, then roll up the tortillas.

*Serving Methods:*

1. Serve with a side of salsa or avocado slices.
2. Wrap in foil for a convenient breakfast on the go.

## Lactose-Free Yogurt and Berry Parfait

*Ingredients:*

- 1 cup lactose-free yogurt

- 1/2 cup mixed berries (e.g., strawberries, blueberries)
- 1/4 cup gluten-free granola
- 1 tablespoon maple syrup

**Preparation Time:** 5 minutes

**Serving Time:** Immediate

**Nutritional Info:** (per serving)

- Calories: 250
- Protein: 10g
- Fiber: 4g

**Instructions:**

- In a glass or bowl, layer lactose-free yogurt with mixed berries.
- Sprinkle gluten-free granola over the yogurt and berries.
- Drizzle with maple syrup for added sweetness.

**Serving Methods:**

1. Garnish with a few fresh mint leaves for a pop of color.
2. Prepare in a mason jar for a portable breakfast option.

## Low FODMAP Banana Pancakes

**Ingredients:**

- 1 ripe banana (under-ripe)
- 2 large eggs
- 1/4 teaspoon cinnamon
- 1 tablespoon maple syrup
- Cooking spray or oil for frying

**Preparation Time:** 10 minutes

**Cooking Time:** 10 minutes

**Serving Time:** Immediate

**Nutritional Info:** (per serving, 2 pancakes)

- Calories: 200
- Protein: 8g
- Fiber: 3g

**Instructions:**

- Mash the ripe banana in a bowl until smooth.
- Add eggs, cinnamon, and maple syrup to the mashed banana. Mix until well combined.
- Heat a non-stick pan over medium heat and lightly coat with cooking spray or oil.
- Pour small portions of the batter onto the pan to form pancakes.
- Cook for 2-3 minutes on each side until golden brown.
- Serve hot with a drizzle of maple syrup.

**Serving Methods:**

1. Top with lactose-free yogurt and fresh berries.
2. Sprinkle with chopped nuts or seeds for added crunch.

## Lactose-Free Scrambled Tofu

*Ingredients:*

- 1/2 block firm tofu, crumbled
- 1/4 cup red bell pepper, diced
- 1/4 cup spinach, chopped
- 1 tablespoon nutritional yeast
- Salt and pepper to taste

*Preparation Time:* 7 minutes

*Cooking Time:* 8 minutes

*Serving Time:* Immediate

*Nutritional Info:* (per serving)

- Calories: 180
- Protein: 12g
- Fiber: 3g

*Instructions:*

- Heat a non-stick skillet over medium heat.
- Add crumbled tofu to the skillet and cook for 3-4 minutes.
- Add diced red bell pepper and chopped spinach to the skillet. Cook until vegetables are tender.

- Sprinkle nutritional yeast over the tofu mixture and season with salt and pepper.
- Continue to cook for another 2-3 minutes, stirring occasionally, until heated through.
- Serve hot.

*Serving Methods:*

1. Wrap the scrambled tofu in a gluten-free tortilla for a breakfast burrito.
2. Serve alongside sliced avocado and cherry tomatoes for a balanced meal.

## Low FODMAP Coconut Berry Smoothie

*Ingredients:*

- 1/2 cup canned coconut milk (unsweetened)
- 1/2 cup mixed berries (e.g., strawberries, raspberries)
- 1 tablespoon chia seeds
- 1 tablespoon shredded coconut (unsweetened)
- Ice cubes

*Preparation Time:* 5 minutes

*Serving Time:* Immediate

*Nutritional Info:* (per serving)

- Calories: 220
- Protein: 4g

- Healthy Fats: 15g

**Instructions:**

- In a blender, combine canned coconut milk, mixed berries, chia seeds, shredded coconut, and ice cubes.
- Blend until smooth.
- Pour into a glass and serve immediately.

**Serving Methods:**

1. Garnish with a few whole berries for a decorative touch.
2. Serve in a chilled coconut bowl for a tropical twist.

# CHAPTER FIVE

## LUNCH RECIPES

## Grilled Chicken Salad with Lemon Vinaigrette

*Ingredients:*

- 2 boneless, skinless chicken breasts
- Mixed salad greens (e.g., spinach, arugula)
- Cherry tomatoes, halved
- Cucumber, sliced
- Red bell pepper, sliced
- Feta cheese, crumbled
- Lemon vinaigrette (lemon juice, olive oil, Dijon mustard, salt)

*Preparation Time:* 10 minutes

*Cooking Time:* 15 minutes

*Serving Time:* 25 minutes

*Nutritional Info:* (per serving)

- Calories: 350
- Protein: 25g
- Healthy Fats: 15g

*Instructions:*

- Season chicken breasts with salt and pepper.
- Grill chicken until fully cooked.
- Slice grilled chicken into strips.

- In a large bowl, combine salad greens, cherry tomatoes, cucumber, red bell pepper, and grilled chicken.
- Top with crumbled feta cheese.
- Drizzle with lemon vinaigrette and toss gently.
- Serve immediately.

**Serving Methods:**

1. Wrap the salad in a gluten-free tortilla for a chicken salad wrap.
2. Serve on a bed of quinoa for a more substantial meal.

# Low FODMAP Quinoa Bowl with Roasted Vegetables

**Ingredients:**

- 1 cup cooked quinoa
- Zucchini, sliced
- Bell peppers, sliced
- Carrots, julienned
- Cherry tomatoes, halved
- Olive oil, for roasting
- Fresh basil, chopped
- Balsamic glaze (optional)

**Preparation Time:** 10 minutes

*Cooking Time:* 20 minutes

*Serving Time:* 30 minutes

*Nutritional Info:* (per serving)

- Calories: 280
- Protein: 8g
- Fiber: 5g

*Instructions:*

- Preheat the oven to 400°F (200°C).
- Toss sliced zucchini, bell peppers, carrots, and cherry tomatoes with olive oil.
- Roast the vegetables in the oven until tender.
- In a bowl, layer cooked quinoa and roasted vegetables.
- Top with fresh basil and drizzle with balsamic glaze if desired.
- Mix gently and serve.

*Serving Methods:*

1. Add grilled chicken or tofu for extra protein.
2. Serve as a cold quinoa salad for a refreshing option.

## Turkey and Cranberry Lettuce Wraps

*Ingredients:*

- 1-pound ground turkey

- Lettuce leaves (e.g., iceberg or butter lettuce)
- Cranberry sauce (without high FODMAP ingredients)
- Shredded carrots
- Walnuts, chopped (optional)
- Salt and pepper to taste

**Preparation Time:** 10 minutes

**Cooking Time:** 15 minutes

**Serving Time:** 25 minutes

**Nutritional Info:** (per serving)

- Calories: 220
- Protein: 18g
- Healthy Fats: 10g

**Instructions:**

- In a skillet, cook ground turkey until browned. Season with salt and pepper.
- Prepare lettuce leaves for wrapping.
- Fill each lettuce leaf with cooked turkey.
- Add shredded carrots and chopped walnuts.
- Drizzle with cranberry sauce.
- Fold the lettuce wraps and secure with toothpicks.
- Serve immediately.

**Serving Methods:**

1. Serve with a side of low FODMAP sweet potato fries.

2. Make it a bowl by skipping the lettuce wraps and serving over rice or quinoa.

# Salmon and Avocado Sushi Bowl

*Ingredients:*

- Cooked sushi rice (follow package instructions)
- Grilled or baked salmon, flaked
- Avocado, sliced
- Cucumber, julienned
- Nori seaweed, shredded
- Gluten-free soy sauce
- Pickled ginger (optional)

*Preparation Time:* 15 minutes

*Cooking Time:* 20 minutes (for rice and salmon)

*Serving Time:* 35 minutes

*Nutritional Info:* (per serving)

- Calories: 320
- Protein: 22g
- Healthy Fats: 15g

*Instructions:*

- Prepare sushi rice according to package instructions.

- In a bowl, layer sushi rice, flaked salmon, sliced avocado, julienned cucumber, and shredded nori seaweed.
- Drizzle with gluten-free soy sauce.
- Garnish with pickled ginger if desired.
- Mix gently and serve.

*Serving Methods:*

1. Make it a sushi burrito by wrapping the ingredients in a sheet of nori.
2. Serve in a hollowed-out bell pepper for a creative and colorful presentation.

# Eggplant and Tomato Stacks

*Ingredients:*

- Eggplant, sliced into rounds
- Tomato, sliced
- Lactose-free mozzarella cheese, sliced
- Fresh basil leaves
- Olive oil
- Balsamic glaze (optional)
- Salt and pepper to taste

*Preparation Time:* 10 minutes

*Cooking Time:* 15 minutes

*Serving Time:* 25 minutes

*Nutritional Info:* (per serving)

- Calories: 180
- Protein: 10g
- Healthy Fats: 8g

*Instructions:*

- Preheat the oven to 375°F (190°C).
- Brush eggplant slices with olive oil and season with salt and pepper.
- Roast the eggplant in the oven until tender.
- Assemble stacks by layering roasted eggplant, sliced tomato, and lactose-free mozzarella.
- Top each stack with fresh basil leaves.
- Drizzle with balsamic glaze if desired.
- Serve warm.

*Serving Methods:*

1. Serve on a bed of spinach for added greens.
2. Accompany with a side of quinoa for a more substantial meal.

## Shrimp and Zoodle Stir-Fry

*Ingredients:*

- Shrimp, peeled and deveined
- Zucchini, spiralized into zoodles
- Red bell pepper, sliced

- Carrots, julienned
- Gluten-free stir-fry sauce
- Sesame oil
- Green onions, chopped (green part only)

**Preparation Time:** 15 minutes

**Cooking Time:** 10 minutes

**Serving Time:** 25 minutes

**Nutritional Info:** (per serving)

- Calories: 220
- Protein: 18g
- Healthy Fats: 8g

**Instructions:**

- In a wok or skillet, heat sesame oil.
- Stir-fry shrimp until pink and cooked through.
- Add zucchini noodles, red bell pepper, and julienned carrots. Cook until vegetables are tender-crisp.
- Pour gluten-free stir-fry sauce over the mixture and toss.
- Garnish with chopped green onions.
- Serve immediately.

**Serving Methods:**

1. Serve over a bed of rice or quinoa.

2. Make it a lettuce wrap by spooning the stir-fry into large lettuce leaves.

## Mediterranean Chickpea Salad

*Ingredients:*

- Canned chickpeas, drained and rinsed
- Cucumber, diced
- Cherry tomatoes, halved
- Kalamata olives, sliced
- Feta cheese, crumbled
- Fresh parsley, chopped
- Olive oil and lemon juice dressing

*Preparation Time:* 10 minutes

*Serving Time:* Immediate

*Nutritional Info:* (per serving)

- Calories: 250
- Protein: 10g
- Healthy Fats: 12g

*Instructions:*

- In a large bowl, combine chickpeas, diced cucumber, cherry tomatoes, sliced Kalamata olives, crumbled feta cheese, and chopped fresh parsley.
- Drizzle with olive oil and lemon juice dressing.

- Toss gently until well combined.
- Serve at room temperature or chilled.

*Serving Methods:*

1. Stuff the salad into bell peppers for a colorful and portable option.
2. Serve over a bed of mixed greens for a heartier meal.

# Chicken and Vegetable Skewers

*Ingredients:*

- Chicken breast, cut into cubes
- Zucchini, sliced
- Bell peppers, cut into chunks
- Cherry tomatoes
- Olive oil
- Garlic-infused oil
- Fresh rosemary, chopped
- Salt and pepper to taste

*Preparation Time:* 15 minutes

*Cooking Time:* 15 minutes

*Serving Time:* 30 minutes

*Nutritional Info:* (per serving)

- Calories: 280
- Protein: 20g

- Healthy Fats: 12g

*Instructions:*

- Preheat the grill or grill pan.
- In a bowl, marinate chicken cubes with olive oil, garlic-infused oil, chopped rosemary, salt, and pepper.
- Thread chicken, zucchini slices, bell pepper chunks, and cherry tomatoes onto skewers.
- Grill until chicken is cooked through and vegetables are tender.
- Serve hot.

*Serving Methods:*

1. Serve over a bed of quinoa or rice.
2. Accompany with a side of low FODMAP tzatziki sauce for dipping.

## Lemon Herb Baked Cod

*Ingredients:*

- Cod fillets
- Lemon, sliced
- Fresh dill, chopped
- Green beans, trimmed
- Olive oil
- Dijon mustard

- Salt and pepper to taste

**Preparation Time:** 10 minutes

**Cooking Time:** 20 minutes

**Serving Time:** 30 minutes

**Nutritional Info:** (per serving)

- Calories: 220
- Protein: 25g
- Healthy Fats: 10g

**Instructions:**

- Preheat the oven to 375°F (190°C).
- In a bowl, mix olive oil, chopped fresh dill, Dijon mustard, salt, and pepper.
- Place cod fillets on a baking sheet.
- Drizzle the olive oil mixture over the cod fillets.
- Top with lemon slices.
- Arrange trimmed green beans around the cod.
- Bake until the fish flakes easily with a fork.
- Serve warm.

**Serving Methods:**

1. Pair with a side of quinoa or roasted sweet potatoes.
2. Serve with a wedge of lemon for additional zesty flavor.

# Lactose-Free Caprese Wrap

## Ingredients:

- Gluten-free tortilla wraps
- Lactose-free mozzarella cheese, sliced
- Tomato, sliced
- Fresh basil leaves
- Balsamic glaze (optional)
- Olive oil
- Salt and pepper to taste

**Preparation Time:** 10 minutes

**Serving Time:** Immediate

**Nutritional Info:** (per serving)

- Calories: 280
- Protein: 12g
- Healthy Fats: 10g

## Instructions:

- Place a lactose-free tortilla on a flat surface.
- Layer with lactose-free mozzarella cheese, tomato slices, and fresh basil leaves.
- Drizzle with olive oil and balsamic glaze if desired.
- Season with salt and pepper to taste.
- Roll up the wrap and slice in half.
- Serve immediately.

## Serving Methods:

1. Pair with a side of mixed greens for a light lunch.

2. Cut into bite-sized pinwheels for a party or snack option.

## Tofu and Vegetable Stir-Fry

*Ingredients:*

- Firm tofu, cubed
- Broccoli florets
- Red bell pepper, sliced
- Carrots, julienned
- Gluten-free stir-fry sauce
- Sesame oil
- Green onions, chopped (green part only)

*Preparation Time:* 15 minutes

*Cooking Time:* 10 minutes

*Serving Time:* 25 minutes

*Nutritional Info:* (per serving)

- Calories: 230
- Protein: 15g
- Healthy Fats: 10g

*Instructions:*

- Press tofu to remove excess water, then cut into cubes.
- In a wok or skillet, heat sesame oil.
- Stir-fry tofu until golden brown.

- Add broccoli florets, sliced red bell pepper, and julienned carrots. Cook until vegetables are tender-crisp.
- Pour gluten-free stir-fry sauce over the mixture and toss.
- Garnish with chopped green onions.
- Serve over rice or quinoa.

*Serving Methods:*
1. Make it a bowl with a base of cooked brown rice.
2. Wrap the stir-fry in lettuce leaves for a low-carb option.

## Low FODMAP Turkey and Vegetable Skillet

*Ingredients:*
- Ground turkey
- Zucchini, diced
- Bell peppers, diced
- Spinach leaves
- Olive oil
- Garlic-infused oil
- Paprika, cumin, salt, and pepper to taste

*Preparation Time:* 10 minutes

*Cooking Time:* 15 minutes

*Serving Time:* 25 minutes

***Nutritional Info:*** (per serving)

- Calories: 240
- Protein: 18g
- Healthy Fats: 10g

***Instructions:***

- In a skillet, heat olive oil and garlic-infused oil.
- Cook ground turkey until browned.
- Add diced zucchini and bell peppers to the skillet. Cook until vegetables are tender.
- Season with paprika, cumin, salt, and pepper.
- Stir in spinach leaves and cook until wilted.
- Serve hot.

***Serving Methods:***

1. Spoon the turkey and vegetable mixture over baked sweet potatoes.
2. Top with a dollop of lactose-free sour cream for added creaminess.

## Low FODMAP Spaghetti with Meat Sauce

***Ingredients:***

- Gluten-free spaghetti
- Ground beef or turkey
- Low FODMAP tomato sauce
- Zucchini, spiralized into zoodles

- Olive oil
- Fresh basil, chopped
- Parmesan cheese (optional)

**Preparation Time:** 15 minutes

**Cooking Time:** 20 minutes

**Serving Time:** 35 minutes

**Nutritional Info:** (per serving)

- Calories: 300
- Protein: 20g
- Healthy Fats: 8g

**Instructions:**

- Cook gluten-free spaghetti according to package instructions.
- In a skillet, brown ground beef or turkey.
- Add low FODMAP tomato sauce and simmer.
- In a separate pan, sauté zucchini noodles in olive oil until tender-crisp.
- Serve spaghetti over zoodles.
- Garnish with chopped fresh basil and Parmesan cheese if desired.

**Serving Methods:**

1. Top with a sprinkle of nutritional yeast for a dairy-free option.

2. Serve with a side of mixed greens dressed in olive oil and lemon juice.

## Lactose-Free Chicken Caesar Salad

*Ingredients:*

- Grilled chicken breast, sliced
- Romaine lettuce, chopped
- Cherry tomatoes, halved
- Lactose-free Caesar dressing
- Gluten-free croutons
- Parmesan cheese (optional)

*Preparation Time:* 10 minutes

*Cooking Time:* 15 minutes (for grilling chicken)

*Serving Time:* 25 minutes

*Nutritional Info:* (per serving)

- Calories: 260
- Protein: 22g
- Healthy Fats: 12g

*Instructions:*

- Grill chicken until fully cooked.
- In a large bowl, combine chopped romaine lettuce and cherry tomatoes.
- Add sliced grilled chicken.

- Drizzle with lactose-free Caesar dressing and toss gently.
- Top with gluten-free croutons and Parmesan cheese if desired.
- Serve immediately.

**Serving Methods:**
1. Roll the salad in a gluten-free tortilla for a chicken Caesar wrap.
2. Serve with a side of roasted sweet potato wedges for added substance.

# Low FODMAP Ratatouille

**Ingredients:**
- Eggplant, diced
- Zucchini, diced
- Bell peppers, diced
- Tomato, diced
- Olive oil
- Garlic-infused oil
- Fresh thyme, chopped
- Salt and pepper to taste

**Preparation Time:** 15 minutes

**Cooking Time:** 25 minutes

**Serving Time:** 40 minutes

***Nutritional Info:*** (per serving)

- Calories: 220
- Protein: 6g
- Healthy Fats: 10g

## *Instructions:*

- In a large skillet, heat olive oil and garlic-infused oil.
- Sauté diced eggplant, zucchini, bell peppers, and tomato until tender.
- Season with fresh thyme, salt, and pepper.
- Continue to cook until flavors meld.
- Serve warm.

## *Serving Methods:*

1. Top with a dollop of lactose-free Greek yogurt for added creaminess.
2. Serve over cooked quinoa or rice for a satisfying meal.

# CHAPTER SIX

# DINNER RECIPES

## Grilled Lemon Herb Chicken

*Ingredients:*

- Chicken thighs or breasts
- Lemon juice
- Olive oil
- Fresh rosemary, chopped
- Fresh thyme, chopped
- Salt and pepper to taste

*Preparation Time:* 10 minutes

*Cooking Time:* 20 minutes

*Serving Time:* 30 minutes

*Nutritional Info:* (per serving)

- Calories: 250
- Protein: 28g
- Healthy Fats: 12g

*Instructions:*

- Preheat the grill or grill pan.
- In a bowl, mix lemon juice, olive oil, chopped rosemary, chopped thyme, salt, and pepper.
- Marinate chicken in the mixture for at least 15 minutes.

- Grill chicken until fully cooked, with nice grill marks.
- Serve hot.

*Serving Methods:*

1. Pair with a side of roasted vegetables.
2. Slice and serve over a bed of quinoa or rice.

# Baked Salmon with Dill Sauce

*Ingredients:*

- Salmon fillets
- Lemon slices
- Fresh dill, chopped
- Olive oil
- Garlic-infused oil
- Dijon mustard
- Salt and pepper to taste

*Preparation Time:* 15 minutes

*Cooking Time:* 15 minutes

*Serving Time:* 30 minutes

*Nutritional Info:* (per serving)

- Calories: 280
- Protein: 25g
- Healthy Fats: 15g

*Instructions:*

- Preheat the oven to 400°F (200°C).
- Place salmon fillets on a baking sheet.
- In a bowl, mix olive oil, garlic-infused oil, chopped fresh dill, Dijon mustard, salt, and pepper.
- Drizzle the mixture over the salmon.
- Top with lemon slices.
- Bake until the salmon is cooked through.
- Serve warm.

*Serving Methods:*

1. Pair with a side of sautéed spinach.
2. Serve over a bed of mashed potatoes for a comforting meal.

# Low FODMAP Turkey and Quinoa Stuffed Peppers

*Ingredients:*

- Bell peppers
- Ground turkey
- Quinoa, cooked
- Zucchini, diced
- Tomato, diced
- Cumin, ground
- Paprika
- Salt and pepper to taste

**Preparation Time:** 15 minutes

**Cooking Time:** 25 minutes

**Serving Time:** 40 minutes

**Nutritional Info:** (per serving)

- Calories: 290
- Protein: 20g
- Fiber: 6g

**Instructions:**

- Preheat the oven to 375°F (190°C).
- Cut the tops off bell peppers and remove seeds.
- In a skillet, cook ground turkey until browned. Add diced zucchini and cook until tender.
- Stir in cooked quinoa, diced tomato, ground cumin, paprika, salt, and pepper.
- Stuff each bell pepper with the turkey and quinoa mixture.
- Bake until peppers are tender.
- Serve hot.

**Serving Methods:**

1. Drizzle with a low FODMAP salsa for added flavor.
2. Top with lactose-free shredded cheese before baking for a cheesy variation.

# Grilled Shrimp and Vegetable Skewers

## Ingredients:

- Shrimp, peeled and deveined
- Zucchini, sliced
- Cherry tomatoes
- Olive oil
- Garlic-infused oil
- Lemon juice
- Fresh parsley, chopped
- Salt and pepper to taste

**Preparation Time:** 15 minutes

**Cooking Time:** 10 minutes

**Serving Time:** 25 minutes

**Nutritional Info:** (per serving)

- Calories: 220
- Protein: 18g
- Healthy Fats: 10g

## Instructions:

- Preheat the grill or grill pan.
- In a bowl, mix olive oil, garlic-infused oil, lemon juice, chopped fresh parsley, salt, and pepper.
- Thread shrimp, zucchini slices, and cherry tomatoes onto skewers.
- Grill until shrimp are pink and cooked through.
- Serve hot.

***Serving Methods:***

1. Serve over a bed of quinoa or rice.
2. Pair with a side of low FODMAP coleslaw for a refreshing option.

# Lemon Garlic Chicken Stir-Fry

***Ingredients:***

- Chicken breast, thinly sliced
- Green beans, trimmed
- Carrots, julienned
- Red bell pepper, sliced
- Gluten-free stir-fry sauce
- Olive oil
- Lemon zest and juice
- Garlic-infused oil
- Salt and pepper to taste

***Preparation Time:*** 15 minutes

***Cooking Time:*** 15 minutes

***Serving Time:*** 30 minutes

***Nutritional Info:*** (per serving)

- Calories: 260
- Protein: 24g
- Healthy Fats: 8g

***Instructions:***

- In a wok or skillet, heat olive oil and garlic-infused oil.
- Stir-fry chicken until browned and cooked through.
- Add trimmed green beans, julienned carrots, and sliced red bell pepper. Cook until vegetables are tender-crisp.
- Pour gluten-free stir-fry sauce over the mixture.
- Add lemon zest and juice.
- Toss until well combined.
- Serve immediately.

**Serving Methods:**
1. Serve over a bed of rice noodles.
2. Pair with a side of steamed jasmine rice.

# Eggplant Lasagna

**Ingredients:**
- Eggplant, thinly sliced lengthwise
- Ground turkey
- Low FODMAP tomato sauce
- Lactose-free mozzarella cheese, shredded
- Fresh basil leaves
- Olive oil
- Salt and pepper to taste

**Preparation Time:** 20 minutes

**Cooking Time:** 30 minutes

**Serving Time:** 50 minutes

**Nutritional Info:** (per serving)

- Calories: 320
- Protein: 22g
- Healthy Fats: 14g

**Instructions:**

- Preheat the oven to 375°F (190°C).
- In a skillet, cook ground turkey until browned. Season with salt and pepper.
- In a baking dish, layer thinly sliced eggplant, cooked ground turkey, and tomato sauce.
- Repeat the layers, finishing with a layer of eggplant on top.
- Top with shredded lactose-free mozzarella cheese.
- Drizzle with olive oil.
- Bake until the cheese is melted and bubbly.
- Garnish with fresh basil leaves.
- Serve warm.

**Serving Methods:**

1. Serve with a side of mixed greens for a balanced meal.

2. Pair with a side of quinoa for added protein and fiber.

# Low FODMAP Teriyaki Chicken

*Ingredients:*

- Chicken thighs or breasts, sliced
- Green beans, trimmed
- Carrots, sliced
- Gluten-free teriyaki sauce
- Sesame oil
- Green onions, chopped (green part only)
- Sesame seeds (optional)
- Brown rice, cooked

*Preparation Time:* 15 minutes

*Cooking Time:* 20 minutes

*Serving Time:* 35 minutes

*Nutritional Info:* (per serving)

- Calories: 310
- Protein: 24g
- Healthy Fats: 10g

*Instructions:*

- In a wok or skillet, heat sesame oil.
- Stir-fry chicken until browned and cooked through.

- Add trimmed green beans and sliced carrots. Cook until vegetables are tender-crisp.
- Pour gluten-free teriyaki sauce over the mixture.
- Stir until well coated.
- Garnish with chopped green onions and sesame seeds if desired.
- Serve over cooked brown rice.

*Serving Methods:*

1. Wrap the teriyaki chicken in lettuce leaves for a low-carb option.
2. Pair with a side of sautéed bok choy for added greens.

## Stuffed Zucchini Boats

*Ingredients:*

- Zucchini, halved lengthwise
- Ground turkey
- Quinoa, cooked
- Low FODMAP tomato sauce
- Lactose-free mozzarella cheese, shredded
- Fresh oregano, chopped
- Olive oil
- Salt and pepper to taste

*Preparation Time:* 20 minutes

*Cooking Time:* 30 minutes

*Serving Time:* 50 minutes

*Nutritional Info:* (per serving)

- Calories: 280
- Protein: 18g
- Healthy Fats: 12g

*Instructions:*

- Preheat the oven to 375°F (190°C).
- Scoop out the center of each zucchini half, creating a "boat."
- In a skillet, cook ground turkey until browned. Season with salt and pepper.
- Stir in cooked quinoa and low FODMAP tomato sauce.
- Spoon the turkey and quinoa mixture into the zucchini boats.
- Top with shredded lactose-free mozzarella cheese and chopped fresh oregano.
- Drizzle with olive oil.
- Bake until zucchini is tender and cheese is melted.
- Serve warm.

*Serving Methods:*

1. Pair with a side of mixed greens for a lighter option.

2. Serve with a side of gluten-free garlic bread for a complete meal.

# Lemon Garlic Shrimp Pasta

*Ingredients:*

- Gluten-free pasta
- Shrimp, peeled and deveined
- Lemon zest and juice
- Garlic-infused oil
- Cherry tomatoes, halved
- Spinach leaves
- Red pepper flakes (optional)
- Fresh parsley, chopped
- Salt and pepper to taste

*Preparation Time:* 15 minutes

*Cooking Time:* 15 minutes

*Serving Time:* 30 minutes

*Nutritional Info:* (per serving)

- Calories: 320
- Protein: 20g
- Healthy Fats: 10g

*Instructions:*

- Cook gluten-free pasta according to package instructions.

- In a skillet, heat garlic-infused oil.
- Add shrimp and cook until pink and cooked through.
- Add lemon zest, lemon juice, halved cherry tomatoes, and spinach leaves.
- Toss until spinach is wilted and tomatoes are softened.
- Season with red pepper flakes, fresh parsley, salt, and pepper.
- Mix in cooked pasta.
- Serve hot.

*Serving Methods:*
1. Sprinkle with grated Parmesan cheese for added flavor.
2. Serve with a side of steamed asparagus for a nutritious addition.

## Low FODMAP Pesto Chicken Skewers

*Ingredients:*
- Chicken breast, cut into cubes
- Cherry tomatoes
- Zucchini, sliced
- Pesto sauce (without high FODMAP ingredients)
- Olive oil

- Salt and pepper to taste

**Preparation Time:** 15 minutes

**Cooking Time:** 15 minutes

**Serving Time:** 30 minutes

**Nutritional Info:** (per serving)

- Calories: 290
- Protein: 22g
- Healthy Fats: 15g

**Instructions:**

- Preheat the grill or grill pan.
- In a bowl, coat chicken cubes with pesto sauce, olive oil, salt, and pepper.
- Thread chicken cubes, cherry tomatoes, and zucchini slices onto skewers.
- Grill until chicken is cooked through and vegetables are tender.
- Serve hot.

**Serving Methods:**

1. Serve over a bed of quinoa or rice.
2. Accompany with a side of roasted sweet potatoes for a satisfying meal.

# Low FODMAP Taco Bowl

**Ingredients:**

- Ground beef or turkey
- Low FODMAP taco seasoning
- Quinoa, cooked
- Lettuce, shredded
- Tomato, diced
- Avocado, sliced
- Salsa (without high FODMAP ingredients)
- Lactose-free sour cream

*Preparation Time:* 15 minutes

*Cooking Time:* 15 minutes

*Serving Time:* 30 minutes

*Nutritional Info:* (per serving)

- Calories: 300
- Protein: 22g
- Fiber: 6g

*Instructions:*

- In a skillet, cook ground beef or turkey until browned. Season with low FODMAP taco seasoning.
- In a bowl, layer cooked quinoa, shredded lettuce, diced tomato, and sliced avocado.
- Top with cooked ground meat.
- Add a dollop of lactose-free sour cream and a spoonful of salsa.

- Serve hot.

*Serving Methods:*

1. Make it a burrito bowl by wrapping the ingredients in a large lettuce leaf.
2. Top with crushed tortilla chips for added crunch.

## Lemon Herb Baked Cod

*Ingredients:*

- Cod fillets
- Lemon, sliced
- Fresh dill, chopped
- Green beans, trimmed
- Olive oil
- Dijon mustard
- Salt and pepper to taste

*Preparation Time:* 10 minutes

*Cooking Time:* 20 minutes

*Serving Time:* 30 minutes

*Nutritional Info:* (per serving)

- Calories: 220
- Protein: 25g
- Healthy Fats: 10g

*Instructions:*

- Preheat the oven to 375°F (190°C).

- In a bowl, mix olive oil, chopped fresh dill, Dijon mustard, salt, and pepper.
- Place cod fillets on a baking sheet.
- Drizzle the olive oil mixture over the cod.
- Top with lemon slices.
- Arrange trimmed green beans around the cod.
- Bake until the fish flakes easily with a fork.
- Serve warm.

*Serving Methods:*

1. Pair with a side of quinoa or roasted sweet potatoes.
2. Serve with a wedge of lemon for additional zesty flavor.

## Low FODMAP Chicken and Vegetable Curry

*Ingredients:*

- Chicken thighs, boneless and skinless, cut into cubes
- Bell peppers, sliced
- Zucchini, sliced
- Carrots, sliced
- Low FODMAP curry paste
- Coconut milk (canned, without high FODMAP ingredients)

- Fresh cilantro, chopped
- Jasmine rice, cooked

**Preparation Time:** 15 minutes

**Cooking Time:** 25 minutes

**Serving Time:** 40 minutes

**Nutritional Info:** (per serving)

- Calories: 330
- Protein: 26g
- Healthy Fats: 15g

**Instructions:**

- In a pot or large skillet, cook chicken until browned.
- Add sliced bell peppers, zucchini, and carrots. Cook until vegetables are tender.
- Stir in low FODMAP curry paste and coconut milk.
- Simmer until the chicken is cooked through and the curry thickens.
- Garnish with chopped fresh cilantro.
- Serve over cooked jasmine rice.

**Serving Methods:**

1. Serve with a side of gluten-free naan bread.
2. Garnish with a wedge of lime for extra zest.

**Low FODMAP Spaghetti Bolognese**

**Ingredients:**

- Ground beef or turkey
- Low FODMAP tomato sauce
- Gluten-free spaghetti
- Olive oil
- Carrots, finely diced
- Fresh basil, chopped
- Parmesan cheese, grated (optional)

**Preparation Time:** 15 minutes

**Cooking Time:** 25 minutes

**Serving Time:** 40 minutes

**Nutritional Info:** (per serving)

- Calories: 280
- Protein: 20g
- Fiber: 5g

**Instructions:**

- In a skillet, cook ground beef or turkey until browned.
- Add finely diced carrots and cook until softened.
- Stir in low FODMAP tomato sauce and fresh basil.
- Simmer until the sauce thickens.
- Cook gluten-free spaghetti according to package instructions.
- Serve the Bolognese sauce over the cooked spaghetti.

- Drizzle with olive oil and sprinkle with grated Parmesan cheese if desired.
- Serve hot.

**Serving Methods:**

1. Make it a low-carb option by serving the Bolognese over zucchini noodles.
2. Garnish with fresh oregano for added flavor.

# Low FODMAP Stir-Fried Tofu with Vegetables

**Ingredients:**

- Firm tofu, cubed
- Broccoli florets
- Snow peas, trimmed
- Red bell pepper, sliced
- Gluten-free soy sauce
- Sesame oil
- Green onions, chopped (green part only)
- Brown rice, cooked

**Preparation Time:** 15 minutes

**Cooking Time:** 15 minutes

**Serving Time:** 30 minutes

**Nutritional Info:** (per serving)

- Calories: 260
- Protein: 18g

- Healthy Fats: 12g

**Instructions:**

- Press tofu to remove excess water, then cut into cubes.
- In a wok or skillet, heat sesame oil.
- Stir-fry tofu until golden brown.
- Add broccoli florets, trimmed snow peas, and sliced red bell pepper. Cook until vegetables are tender-crisp.
- Pour gluten-free soy sauce over the mixture and toss.
- Garnish with chopped green onions.
- Serve over cooked brown rice.

**Serving Methods:**

1. Make it a low-carb option by serving the stir-fry over cauliflower rice.
2. Drizzle with a little chili oil for a spicy kick.

## Greek Yogurt Parfait

*Ingredients:*

- Lactose-free Greek yogurt
- Strawberries, sliced
- Blueberries
- Gluten-free granola
- Maple syrup (optional)

*Preparation Time:* 5 minutes

*Serving Time:* Immediate

*Nutritional Info:* (per serving)

- Calories: 180
- Protein: 10g
- Fiber: 4g

*Instructions:*

- In a glass or bowl, layer lactose-free Greek yogurt, sliced strawberries, blueberries, and gluten-free granola.
- Repeat the layers.
- Drizzle with maple syrup if desired.
- Serve chilled.

*Serving Methods:*

1. Top with a dollop of almond butter for added creaminess.

2. Garnish with mint leaves for a refreshing touch.

# Rice Cake with Almond Butter and Banana Slices

*Ingredients:*

- Rice cakes
- Almond butter
- Banana, sliced
- Chia seeds

*Preparation Time:* 5 minutes

*Serving Time:* Immediate

*Nutritional Info:* (per serving)

- Calories: 150
- Protein: 5g
- Healthy Fats: 8g

*Instructions:*

- Spread almond butter on a rice cake.
- Top with banana slices.
- Sprinkle chia seeds over the top.
- Serve as an open-faced snack.

*Serving Methods:*

1. Make it a sandwich by adding another rice cake on top.
2. Drizzle with a touch of honey for sweetness.

## Cucumber and Hummus Bites

*Ingredients:*
- Cucumber, sliced
- Low FODMAP hummus
- Cherry tomatoes, halved
- Fresh dill, chopped

*Preparation Time:* 10 minutes

*Serving Time:* Immediate

*Nutritional Info:* (per serving)
- Calories: 70
- Protein: 3g
- Fiber: 2g

*Instructions:*
- Place cucumber slices on a serving platter.
- Spoon a small amount of low FODMAP hummus onto each cucumber slice.
- Top with a halved cherry tomato.
- Garnish with chopped fresh dill.
- Serve chilled.

*Serving Methods:*

1. Add a sprinkle of black pepper for extra flavor.
2. Use zucchini slices as an alternative to cucumber.

## Hard-Boiled Eggs with Paprika

*Ingredients:*

- Hard-boiled eggs
- Paprika
- Salt and pepper to taste
- Fresh chives, chopped

*Preparation Time:* 10 minutes

*Cooking Time:* 10 minutes (for boiling)

*Serving Time:* Immediate

*Nutritional Info:* (per serving)

- Calories: 70
- Protein: 6g
- Healthy Fats: 5g

*Instructions:*

- Peel hard-boiled eggs and cut them in half.
- Sprinkle paprika, salt, and pepper over each egg half.
- Garnish with chopped fresh chives.
- Serve chilled.

*Serving Methods:*

1. Place each egg half on a slice of cucumber for a crunchy base.
2. Drizzle with a touch of olive oil for added richness.

## Trail Mix with Nuts and Seeds

*Ingredients:*

- Mixed nuts (almonds, walnuts, and pecans)
- Pumpkin seeds
- Sunflower seeds
- Dried cranberries (in moderation)
- Dark chocolate chips (optional)

*Preparation Time:* 5 minutes

*Serving Time:* Immediate

*Nutritional Info:* (per serving)

- Calories: 200
- Protein: 6g
- Healthy Fats: 15g

*Instructions:*

- In a bowl, mix together mixed nuts, pumpkin seeds, sunflower seeds, and dried cranberries.
- Add dark chocolate chips if desired.
- Toss to combine.
- Serve in small portions.

*Serving Methods:*

1. Pair with lactose-free yogurt for a more filling snack.
2. Pack in individual snack-sized bags for on-the-go.

## Low FODMAP Caprese Skewers

*Ingredients:*

- Cherry tomatoes
- Lactose-free mozzarella balls
- Basil leaves
- Balsamic glaze (optional)

*Preparation Time:* 10 minutes

*Serving Time:* Immediate

*Nutritional Info:* (per serving)

- Calories: 120
- Protein: 5g
- Healthy Fats: 8g

*Instructions:*

- Thread a cherry tomato, a mozzarella ball, and a basil leaf onto small skewers.
- Repeat for each skewer.
- Arrange on a serving platter.
- Drizzle with balsamic glaze if desired.
- Serve at room temperature.

*Serving Methods:*

1. Arrange on a bed of arugula for a more substantial salad.
2. Serve with a side of gluten-free crackers.

## Low FODMAP Fruit Salad

*Ingredients:*

- Strawberries, hulled and halved
- Blueberries
- Kiwi, peeled and sliced
- Pineapple, diced
- Mint leaves, chopped
- Lime juice

*Preparation Time:* 10 minutes

*Serving Time:* Immediate

*Nutritional Info:* (per serving)

- Calories: 80
- Fiber: 3g
- Vitamin C: 70% DV

*Instructions:*

- In a bowl, combine strawberries, blueberries, sliced kiwi, and diced pineapple.
- Drizzle with fresh lime juice.
- Sprinkle chopped mint leaves over the top.
- Gently toss to combine.

- Serve chilled.

*Serving Methods:*

- Top with a dollop of lactose-free whipped cream for a treat.

- Mix in a handful of toasted coconut for added texture.

## Low FODMAP Guacamole with Veggie Sticks

*Ingredients:*

- Avocado, mashed
- Tomato, diced
- Cilantro, chopped
- Lime juice
- Salt and pepper to taste
- Carrot and bell pepper sticks

*Preparation Time:* 10 minutes

*Serving Time:* Immediate

*Nutritional Info:* (per serving)

- Calories: 100
- Healthy Fats: 8g
- Fiber: 5g

*Instructions:*

- In a bowl, mash avocado and mix with diced tomato, chopped cilantro, lime juice, salt, and pepper.
- Stir until well combined.
- Serve with carrot and bell pepper sticks for dipping.
- Serve chilled.

*Serving Methods:*

1. Pair with gluten-free tortilla chips for a heartier snack.
2. Spread on rice cakes for a quick and tasty alternative.

# Baked Zucchini Chips

*Ingredients:*

- Zucchini, thinly sliced
- Olive oil
- Paprika
- Garlic-infused oil
- Salt and pepper to taste

*Preparation Time:* 10 minutes

*Cooking Time:* 20 minutes

*Serving Time:* Immediate

*Nutritional Info:* (per serving)

- Calories: 90
- Fiber: 3g
- Vitamin C: 20% DV

*Instructions:*

- Preheat the oven to 400°F (200°C).
- Toss thinly sliced zucchini with olive oil, paprika, garlic-infused oil, salt, and pepper.
- Arrange slices on a baking sheet in a single layer.
- Bake until golden and crispy.
- Serve immediately.

*Serving Methods:*

1. Dip in a low FODMAP tzatziki sauce for added flavor.
2. Sprinkle with nutritional yeast for a cheesy twist.

## Lactose-Free Cottage Cheese with Pineapple

*Ingredients:*

- Lactose-free cottage cheese
- Fresh pineapple, diced
- Chia seeds
- Honey (optional)

*Preparation Time:* 5 minutes

*Serving Time:* Immediate

*Nutritional Info:* (per serving)

- Calories: 120
- Protein: 10g
- Fiber: 2g

*Instructions:*

- In a bowl, combine lactose-free cottage cheese and diced fresh pineapple.
- Sprinkle chia seeds over the top.
- Drizzle with honey if desired.
- Serve chilled.

*Serving Methods:*

1. Top with a handful of gluten-free granola for added crunch.
2. Mix in a few fresh mint leaves for a burst of freshness.

# Lemon Herb Rice Crackers with Smoked Salmon

*Ingredients:*

- Rice crackers
- Smoked salmon
- Lemon zest
- Fresh dill, chopped
- Dairy-free cream cheese

*Preparation Time:* 10 minutes

*Serving Time:* Immediate

*Nutritional Info:* (per serving)

- Calories: 110
- Protein: 5g
- Healthy Fats: 7g

**Instructions:**

- Spread dairy-free cream cheese on rice crackers.
- Top with smoked salmon.
- Sprinkle lemon zest and chopped fresh dill over each cracker.
- Serve immediately.

*Serving Methods:*

1. Garnish with capers for a briny kick.
2. Serve with a side of arugula for a light salad.

# Low FODMAP Chocolate Banana Bites

*Ingredients:*

- Banana, sliced
- Dark chocolate, melted
- Almond butter
- Chopped nuts (walnuts or almonds)

*Preparation Time:* 10 minutes

*Serving Time:* Immediate

*Nutritional Info:* (per serving)

- Calories: 130
- Healthy Fats: 8g
- Fiber: 3g

**Instructions:**

- Dip banana slices in melted dark chocolate.
- Drizzle with almond butter.
- Sprinkle chopped nuts over each banana bite.
- Place on a tray and let the chocolate set.
- Serve chilled.

**Serving Methods:**

1. Freeze for a cool and refreshing treat.
2. Pair with a scoop of lactose-free vanilla ice cream.

## Low FODMAP Sushi Rolls

**Ingredients:**

- Nori sheets
- Cooked and cooled sushi rice
- Sliced cucumber
- Carrot matchsticks
- Cooked shrimp or crab (if tolerated)
- Gluten-free soy sauce (tamari)

**Preparation Time:** 15 minutes

**Serving Time:** Immediate

**Nutritional Info:** (per serving)

- Calories: 160
- Protein: 5g
- Fiber: 2g

**Instructions:**

- Place a nori sheet on a bamboo sushi mat.
- Spread a thin layer of sushi rice over the nori.
- Arrange sliced cucumber, carrot matchsticks, and cooked shrimp or crab along one edge.
- Roll tightly using the sushi mat.
- Slice into bite-sized pieces.
- Serve with gluten-free soy sauce for dipping.

**Serving Methods:**

1. Add a layer of avocado for extra creaminess.
2. Serve with pickled ginger and wasabi for traditional sushi accompaniments.

# Low FODMAP Berry Smoothie Bowl

**Ingredients:**

- Mixed berries (strawberries, blueberries, raspberries)
- Lactose-free yogurt
- Banana (use in moderation)
- Chia seeds
- Gluten-free granola

**Preparation Time:** 10 minutes

**Serving Time:** Immediate

**Nutritional Info:** (per serving)

- Calories: 180
- Protein: 6g
- Fiber: 5g

**Instructions:**

- Blend mixed berries, lactose-free yogurt, and a small amount of banana until smooth.
- Pour into a bowl.
- Top with chia seeds and gluten-free granola.
- Serve immediately.

**Serving Methods:**

1. Add a spoonful of almond butter for extra richness.
2. Garnish with fresh mint leaves for a burst of flavor.

# Low FODMAP Energy Bites

**Ingredients:**

- Rolled oats
- Almond butter
- Chia seeds
- Dark chocolate chips
- Maple syrup
- Vanilla extract

*Preparation Time:* 10 minutes

*Chilling Time:* 30 minutes

*Serving Time*: Immediate

*Nutritional Info:* (per serving, 2 bites)

- Calories: 120
- Protein: 4g
- Healthy Fats: 6g

*Instructions:*

- In a bowl, mix rolled oats, almond butter, chia seeds, dark chocolate chips, maple syrup, and vanilla extract.
- Roll into bite-sized balls.
- Place in the refrigerator to chill.
- Serve cold.

*Serving Methods:*

1. Dust with a little cocoa powder for a chocolatey finish.
2. Store in an airtight container for a convenient grab-and-go snack.

# CHAPTER EIGHT

# DESSERT RECIPES

## Strawberry Almond Chia Pudding

*Ingredients:*

- Lactose-free almond milk
- Chia seeds
- Strawberries, sliced
- Maple syrup
- Almonds, chopped

*Preparation Time:* 10 minutes

*Chilling Time:* 4 hours or overnight

*Serving Time:* Immediate

*Nutritional Info:* (per serving)

- Calories: 150
- Fiber: 6g
- Healthy Fats: 8g

*Instructions:*

- Mix chia seeds with lactose-free almond milk in a bowl.
- Add sliced strawberries, maple syrup, and chopped almonds.
- Stir well and refrigerate until set.

- Serve chilled.

*Serving Methods:*

1. Top with a dollop of lactose-free whipped cream.
2. Garnish with fresh mint leaves for a vibrant touch.

# Low FODMAP Chocolate Avocado Mousse

*Ingredients:*

- Ripe avocados
- Cocoa powder
- Maple syrup
- Vanilla extract
- Lactose-free coconut milk

*Preparation Time:* 15 minutes

*Chilling Time:* 2 hours

*Serving Time:* Immediate

*Nutritional Info:* (per serving)

- Calories: 180
- Fiber: 5g
- Healthy Fats: 12g

*Instructions:*

- Blend avocados, cocoa powder, maple syrup, vanilla extract, and lactose-free coconut milk until smooth.
- Refrigerate until chilled.

- Serve in individual bowls.

***Serving Methods:***

1. Top with shaved dark chocolate for extra decadence.
2. Serve with a side of fresh berries for a fruity contrast.

# Low FODMAP Lemon Poppy Seed Muffins

***Ingredients:***

- Gluten-free flour
- Baking powder
- Lemon zest
- Poppy seeds
- Lactose-free butter
- Maple syrup
- Eggs

***Preparation Time:*** 15 minutes

***Baking Time:*** 20 minutes

***Serving Time:*** Immediate

***Nutritional Info:*** (per serving)

- Calories: 160
- Protein: 4g
- Healthy Fats: 7g

***Instructions:***

- Preheat the oven to 350°F (175°C).
- Mix gluten-free flour, baking powder, lemon zest, and poppy seeds in a bowl.
- In a separate bowl, cream lactose-free butter and maple syrup. Add eggs one at a time.
- Combine wet and dry ingredients.
- Spoon batter into muffin cups and bake until golden.

*Serving Methods:*

1. Dust with powdered sugar for a sweet finish.
2. Serve with a side of lactose-free yogurt for added creaminess.

## Low FODMAP Berry Crisp

*Ingredients:*

- Mixed berries (strawberries, blueberries, raspberries)
- Gluten-free oats
- Almond flour
- Maple syrup
- Lactose-free butter

*Preparation Time:* 15 minutes

*Baking Time:* 30 minutes

*Serving Time:* Immediate

***Nutritional Info:*** (per serving)

- Calories: 180
- Fiber: 5g
- Healthy Fats: 9g

***Instructions:***

- Preheat the oven to 375°F (190°C).
- Mix mixed berries with maple syrup and place in a baking dish.
- In a separate bowl, combine gluten-free oats, almond flour, and melted lactose-free butter.
- Spread the oat mixture over the berries.
- Bake until golden and bubbly.

***Serving Methods:***

1. Top with a scoop of lactose-free vanilla ice cream.
2. Serve with a drizzle of warm low FODMAP chocolate sauce.

## Low FODMAP Vanilla Coconut Panna Cotta

***Ingredients:***

- Lactose-free coconut milk
- Gelatin
- Maple syrup
- Vanilla extract

***Preparation Time:*** 10 minutes

*Chilling Time:* 4 hours or overnight

*Serving Time:* Immediate

*Nutritional Info:* (per serving)

- Calories: 120
- Protein: 3g
- Healthy Fats: 8g

*Instructions:*

- Heat lactose-free coconut milk until warm but not boiling.
- Dissolve gelatin in the milk.
- Add maple syrup and vanilla extract. Mix well.
- Pour into molds and refrigerate until set.
- Serve chilled.

*Serving Methods:*

1. Top with fresh berries for a burst of flavor.
2. Garnish with toasted coconut for added texture.

# Low FODMAP Cinnamon Baked Apples

*Ingredients:*

- Apples, cored and sliced
- Cinnamon
- Maple syrup
- Lactose-free butter

*Preparation Time:* 10 minutes

**Baking Time:** 25 minutes

**Serving Time:** Immediate

**Nutritional Info:** (per serving)

- Calories: 90
- Fiber: 4g
- Healthy Fats: 4g

**Instructions:**

- Preheat the oven to 375°F (190°C).
- Toss apple slices with cinnamon and maple syrup.
- Place in a baking dish and dot with lactose-free butter.
- Bake until apples are tender.

**Serving Methods:**

1. Serve with a scoop of lactose-free vanilla yogurt.
2. Top with a sprinkle of chopped nuts for added crunch.

# Low FODMAP Pumpkin Spice Energy Balls

**Ingredients:**

- Pumpkin puree
- Rolled oats
- Almond butter
- Pumpkin spice
- Maple syrup

- Chopped pecans

**Preparation Time:** 15 minutes

**Chilling Time:** 30 minutes

**Serving Time:** Immediate

**Nutritional Info:** (per serving, 2 balls)

- Calories: 110
- Protein: 3g
- Healthy Fats: 6g

**Instructions:**

- In a bowl, mix pumpkin puree, rolled oats, almond butter, pumpkin spice, maple syrup, and chopped pecans.
- Roll into bite-sized balls.
- Chill in the refrigerator.
- Serve cold.

**Serving Methods:**

1. Roll in shredded coconut for a tropical twist.
2. Drizzle with a touch of honey before serving.

## Low FODMAP Chocolate Dipped Strawberries

**Ingredients:**

- Strawberries, washed and dried
- Dark chocolate, melted

**Preparation Time:** 10 minutes

**Chilling Time:** 30 minutes

**Serving Time:** Immediate

**Nutritional Info:** (per serving)

- Calories: 70
- Fiber: 2g
- Healthy Fats: 4g

**Instructions:**

- Dip each strawberry into melted dark chocolate.
- Place on a tray lined with parchment paper.
- Chill until the chocolate sets.

**Serving Methods:**

1. Drizzle with a little melted white chocolate for a decorative touch.
2. Crushed nuts can be sprinkled over the chocolate for added crunch.

# Low FODMAP Coconut Rice Pudding

**Ingredients:**

- Arborio rice
- Lactose-free coconut milk
- Maple syrup
- Shredded coconut
- Vanilla extract

**Preparation Time:** 10 minutes

*Cooking Time:* 25 minutes

*Serving Time:* Immediate

*Nutritional Info:* (per serving)

- Calories: 160
- Protein: 2g
- Healthy Fats: 7g

*Instructions:*

- Cook Arborio rice in lactose-free coconut milk until tender.
- Stir in maple syrup, shredded coconut, and vanilla extract.
- Cook until the mixture thickens.
- Serve warm.

*Serving Methods:*

1. Sprinkle ground cinnamon over the top for a warm flavor.
2. Top with a dollop of lactose-free whipped cream.

## Low FODMAP Blueberry Oat Bars

*Ingredients:*

- Gluten-free oats
- Blueberries
- Maple syrup
- Almond flour

- Lactose-free butter

**Preparation Time:** 15 minutes

**Baking Time:** 30 minutes

**Serving Time:** Immediate

**Nutritional Info:** (per serving)

- Calories: 120
- Fiber: 3g
- Healthy Fats: 6g

**Instructions:**

- Preheat the oven to 350°F (175°C).
- Mix gluten-free oats, blueberries, maple syrup, almond flour, and melted lactose-free butter.
- Press into a baking dish and bake until golden.
- Allow to cool before slicing.

**Serving Methods:**

1. Serve with a scoop of lactose-free vanilla ice cream.
2. Drizzle with low FODMAP caramel sauce for added sweetness.

## Low FODMAP Raspberry Sorbet

**Ingredients:**

- Raspberries
- Maple syrup

- Lemon juice

*Preparation Time:* 10 minutes

*Freezing Time:* 4 hours or overnight

*Serving Time:* Immediate

*Nutritional Info:* (per serving)

- Calories: 60
- Fiber: 4g
- Vitamin C: 40% DV

*Instructions:*

- Blend raspberries, maple syrup, and lemon juice until smooth.
- Pour into a shallow dish and freeze.
- Scrape with a fork to create a sorbet texture.
- Serve immediately.

*Serving Methods:*

1. Garnish with fresh mint leaves for a burst of freshness.
2. Serve in a chilled glass for an elegant presentation.

## Low FODMAP Chocolate Banana Ice Cream

*Ingredients:*

- Bananas, sliced and frozen
- Cocoa powder

- Almond milk

**Preparation Time:** 5 minutes

**Freezing Time:** 4 hours or overnight

**Serving Time:** Immediate

**Nutritional Info:** (per serving)

- Calories: 100
- Fiber: 3g
- Healthy Fats: 2g

**Instructions:**

- Blend frozen banana slices, cocoa powder, and almond milk until creamy.
- Freeze until firm.
- Serve as scoops.

**Serving Methods:**

1. Top with chopped nuts for added texture.
2. Drizzle with low FODMAP chocolate sauce for a decadent finish.

# Low FODMAP Almond Butter Cookies

**Ingredients:**

- Almond flour
- Almond butter
- Maple syrup
- Vanilla extract

*Preparation Time:* 10 minutes

*Baking Time:* 12 minutes

*Serving Time:* Immediate

*Nutritional Info:* (per serving, 2 cookies)

- Calories: 120
- Protein: 4g
- Healthy Fats: 9g

*Instructions:*

- Preheat the oven to 350°F (175°C).
- Mix almond flour, almond butter, maple syrup, and vanilla extract.
- Form into small cookies and bake until golden.
- Allow to cool before serving.

*Serving Methods:*

1. Sandwich two cookies with a layer of lactose-free vanilla frosting.
2. Sprinkle with a pinch of sea salt for a sweet and salty combination.

## Low FODMAP Peanut Butter Banana Bites

*Ingredients:*

- Bananas, sliced
- Peanut butter
- Dark chocolate, melted

- Chopped peanuts

**Preparation Time:** 10 minutes

**Chilling Time:** 30 minutes

**Serving Time:** Immediate

**Nutritional Info:** (per serving)

- Calories: 80
- Protein: 2g
- Healthy Fats: 5g

**Instructions:**

- Spread peanut butter on banana slices.
- Dip each slice into melted dark chocolate.
- Sprinkle with chopped peanuts.
- Chill until the chocolate sets.

**Serving Methods:**

1. Freeze for a refreshing treat.
2. Serve with a side of low FODMAP fruit compote.

# Low FODMAP Mango Sorbet

**Ingredients:**

- Mango, peeled and diced
- Maple syrup
- Lime juice

**Preparation Time:** 10 minutes

**Freezing Time:** 4 hours or overnight

***Serving Time:*** Immediate

***Nutritional Info:*** (per serving)

- Calories: 70
- Fiber: 2g
- Vitamin C: 60% DV

***Instructions:***

- Blend mango, maple syrup, and lime juice until smooth.
- Freeze in a shallow dish.
- Scoop and serve immediately.

***Serving Methods:***

1. Garnish with a slice of lime for a citrusy touch.
2. Serve in a hollowed-out half of a fresh mango for a creative presentation.

# CHAPTER NINE

# SALAD RECIPES

## Low FODMAP Greek Salad

*Ingredients:*

- Cucumber, diced
- Cherry tomatoes, halved
- Kalamata olives, pitted
- Feta cheese, crumbled
- Olive oil
- Lemon juice
- Fresh oregano, chopped

*Preparation Time:* 10 minutes

*Serving Time:* Immediate

*Nutritional Info:* (per serving)

- Calories: 120
- Protein: 4g
- Healthy Fats: 10g

*Instructions:*

- In a bowl, combine cucumber, cherry tomatoes, Kalamata olives, and feta cheese.
- Drizzle with olive oil and lemon juice.
- Sprinkle with fresh oregano.
- Toss gently to combine.

- Serve chilled.

1. Top with grilled chicken for a protein boost.
2. Serve over a bed of spinach for added greens.

## Low FODMAP Quinoa Salad with Roasted Vegetables

*Ingredients:*

- Quinoa, cooked
- Zucchini, diced
- Bell peppers, sliced
- Cherry tomatoes, halved
- Olive oil
- Balsamic vinegar
- Fresh basil, chopped

*Preparation Time:* 15 minutes

*Cooking Time:* 20 minutes (for roasting)

*Serving Time:* Immediate

*Nutritional Info:* (per serving)

- Calories: 180
- Protein: 5g
- Fiber: 4g

*Instructions:*

- Toss diced zucchini, sliced bell peppers, and cherry tomatoes with olive oil.
- Roast until vegetables are tender.
- Mix roasted vegetables with cooked quinoa.
- Drizzle with balsamic vinegar and sprinkle with fresh basil.
- Serve at room temperature.

*Serving Methods:*
1. Top with crumbled feta for added creaminess.
2. Serve over a bed of arugula for a peppery twist.

## Low FODMAP Chicken Caesar Salad

*Ingredients:*
- Grilled chicken breast, sliced
- Romaine lettuce, chopped
- Parmesan cheese, shaved
- Gluten-free croutons
- Caesar dressing (low FODMAP)

*Preparation Time:* 15 minutes

*Cooking Time:* 15 minutes (for grilling chicken, if not pre-cooked)

*Serving Time:* Immediate

*Nutritional Info:* (per serving)
- Calories: 220

- Protein: 20g
- Healthy Fats: 12g

**Instructions:**

- Grill chicken breast until cooked through, then slice.
- In a large bowl, combine chopped romaine lettuce, sliced grilled chicken, shaved Parmesan, and gluten-free croutons.
- Drizzle with low FODMAP Caesar dressing.
- Toss gently to coat.
- Serve immediately.

**Serving Methods:**

1. Substitute chicken with grilled shrimp for a seafood twist.
2. Add cherry tomatoes for extra freshness.

## Low FODMAP Caprese Salad

**Ingredients:**

- Tomatoes, sliced
- Lactose-free mozzarella balls
- Fresh basil leaves
- Balsamic glaze
- Olive oil
- Salt and pepper to taste

***Preparation Time:*** 10 minutes

***Serving Time:*** Immediate

***Nutritional Info:*** (per serving)

- Calories: 140
- Protein: 8g
- Healthy Fats: 10g

***Instructions:***

- Arrange tomato slices, lactose-free mozzarella balls, and fresh basil leaves on a serving platter.
- Drizzle with balsamic glaze and olive oil.
- Sprinkle with salt and pepper to taste.
- Serve at room temperature.

***Serving Methods:***

1. Top with chopped roasted nuts for added crunch.
2. Serve with gluten-free crackers for a light appetizer.

## Low FODMAP Spinach and Strawberry Salad

***Ingredients:***

- Baby spinach leaves
- Strawberries, sliced
- Feta cheese, crumbled
- Walnuts, chopped
- Olive oil

- Balsamic vinegar

**Preparation Time:** 10 minutes

**Serving Time:** Immediate

**Nutritional Info:** (per serving)

- Calories: 150
- Protein: 4g
- Healthy Fats: 12g

**Instructions:**

- In a bowl, combine baby spinach, sliced strawberries, crumbled feta, and chopped walnuts.
- Drizzle with olive oil and balsamic vinegar.
- Toss gently to combine.
- Serve chilled.

**Serving Methods:**

1. Add grilled chicken for a complete meal.
2. Substitute feta with lactose-free goat cheese.

## Low FODMAP Asian-Inspired Cucumber Salad

**Ingredients:**

- English cucumber, thinly sliced
- Carrots, julienned
- Red bell pepper, thinly sliced
- Green onions, chopped (green parts only)

- Sesame seeds
- Rice vinegar
- Tamari (gluten-free soy sauce)

Preparation Time: 10 minutes

Serving Time: Immediate

Nutritional Info: (per serving)

- Calories: 80
- Fiber: 2g
- Vitamin C: 30% DV

## Instructions:

- In a bowl, combine thinly sliced cucumber, julienned carrots, sliced red bell pepper, and chopped green onions.
- Drizzle with rice vinegar and tamari.
- Sprinkle with sesame seeds.
- Toss gently to coat.
- Serve at room temperature.

## Serving Methods:

1. Add grilled shrimp or tofu for a protein boost.
2. Serve over a bed of quinoa for a heartier dish.

# Low FODMAP Tuna Salad with Green Beans

## Ingredients:

- Canned tuna, drained

- Green beans, blanched and cut into bite-sized pieces
- Cherry tomatoes, halved
- Black olives, pitted and sliced
- Olive oil
- Lemon juice
- Dijon mustard

**Preparation Time:** 15 minutes

**Cooking Time:** 5 minutes (for blanching green beans)

**Serving Time:** Immediate

**Nutritional Info:** (per serving)

- Calories: 180
- Protein: 15g
- Healthy Fats: 10g

**Instructions:**

- In a bowl, combine drained tuna, blanched green beans, cherry tomatoes, and sliced black olives.
- In a separate small bowl, whisk together olive oil, lemon juice, and Dijon mustard to make the dressing.
- Pour the dressing over the salad and toss gently.
- Serve chilled.

**Serving Methods:**

1. Add boiled baby potatoes for a more substantial meal.
2. Top with a sprinkle of fresh parsley for a burst of flavor.

## Low FODMAP Waldorf Salad

*Ingredients:*

- Apples, diced
- Grapes, halved
- Celery, thinly sliced
- Walnuts, chopped
- Lactose-free mayonnaise
- Lemon juice

*Preparation Time:* 10 minutes

*Serving Time:* Immediate

*Nutritional Info:* (per serving)

- Calories: 160
- Fiber: 3g
- Healthy Fats: 10g

*Instructions:*

- In a bowl, combine diced apples, halved grapes, thinly sliced celery, and chopped walnuts.
- In a small bowl, mix lactose-free mayonnaise and a splash of lemon juice to create the dressing.

- Pour the dressing over the salad and toss gently.
- Serve chilled.

**Serving Methods:**

1. Add grilled chicken or turkey for a protein-rich salad.
2. Serve on a bed of mixed greens for added variety.

# Low FODMAP Spinach and Bacon Salad

*Ingredients:*

- Baby spinach leaves
- Cooked bacon, crumbled
- Cherry tomatoes, halved
- Hard-boiled eggs, sliced
- Dijon mustard vinaigrette

*Preparation Time:* 15 minutes

*Cooking Time:* 10 minutes (for bacon and eggs)

*Serving Time:* Immediate

*Nutritional Info:* (per serving)

- Calories: 190
- Protein: 8g
- Healthy Fats: 12g

*Instructions:*

- In a bowl, combine baby spinach, crumbled bacon, halved cherry tomatoes, and sliced hard-boiled eggs.
- Drizzle with Dijon mustard vinaigrette.
- Toss gently to combine.
- Serve at room temperature.

*Serving Methods:*

1. Top with crumbled feta or blue cheese for added richness.
2. Add avocado slices for a creamy texture.

# Low FODMAP Mediterranean Chickpea Salad

*Ingredients:*

- Chickpeas, drained and rinsed
- Cucumber, diced
- Cherry tomatoes, halved
- Red onion, finely chopped
- Feta cheese, crumbled
- Kalamata olives, pitted and sliced
- Olive oil
- Red wine vinegar
- Fresh parsley, chopped

*Preparation Time:* 15 minutes

*Serving Time:* Immediate

***Nutritional Info:*** (per serving)

- Calories: 180
- Protein: 6g
- Healthy Fats: 10g

***Instructions:***

- In a bowl, combine chickpeas, diced cucumber, halved cherry tomatoes, finely chopped red onion, crumbled feta, and sliced Kalamata olives.
- Drizzle with olive oil and red wine vinegar.
- Sprinkle with fresh parsley.
- Toss gently to combine.
- Serve chilled.

***Serving Methods:***

1. Add grilled chicken or shrimp for a protein-packed meal.
2. Serve over a bed of quinoa or rice for a more substantial dish.

## Low FODMAP Shrimp and Avocado Salad

***Ingredients:***

- Shrimp, cooked and peeled
- Avocado, diced
- Grapefruit segments
- Mixed salad greens

- Olive oil
- Lime juice
- Dijon mustard

**Preparation Time:** 15 minutes

**Cooking Time:** 5 minutes (for cooking shrimp, if not pre-cooked)

**Serving Time:** Immediate

**Nutritional Info:** (per serving)

- Calories: 160
- Protein: 10g
- Healthy Fats: 8g

**Instructions:**

- In a bowl, combine cooked shrimp, diced avocado, grapefruit segments, and mixed salad greens.
- In a small bowl, whisk together olive oil, lime juice, and Dijon mustard to make the dressing.
- Pour the dressing over the salad and toss gently.
- Serve at room temperature.

**Serving Methods:**

1. Top with a sprinkle of chia seeds for added nutrition.
2. Serve with a side of gluten-free bread for a complete meal.

# Low FODMAP Roasted Vegetable Salad

## Ingredients:

- Mixed baby greens
- Roasted sweet potatoes, diced
- Roasted carrots, sliced
- Roasted red bell peppers, sliced
- Goat cheese, crumbled
- Balsamic vinaigrette

**Preparation Time:** 15 minutes

**Cooking Time:** 30 minutes (for roasting vegetables)

**Serving Time:** Immediate

**Nutritional Info:** (per serving)

- Calories: 170
- Fiber: 4g
- Healthy Fats: 9g

## Instructions:

- In a bowl, combine mixed baby greens, diced roasted sweet potatoes, sliced roasted carrots, sliced roasted red bell peppers, and crumbled goat cheese.
- Drizzle with balsamic vinaigrette.
- Toss gently to combine.
- Serve at room temperature.

## Serving Methods:

1. Top with grilled chicken or salmon for added protein.
2. Sprinkle with toasted pumpkin seeds for a crunchy texture.

## Low FODMAP Tofu and Vegetable Noodle Salad

*Ingredients:*

- Rice noodles, cooked
- Extra-firm tofu, cubed and pan-fried
- Cucumber, julienned
- Carrots, julienned
- Red bell pepper, thinly sliced
- Green onions, chopped (green parts only)
- Sesame oil
- Tamari (gluten-free soy sauce)
- Sesame seeds

*Preparation Time:* 20 minutes

*Cooking Time:* 15 minutes (for pan-frying tofu and cooking noodles)

*Serving Time:* Immediate

*Nutritional Info:* (per serving)

- Calories: 190
- Protein: 8g

- Healthy Fats: 6g

**Instructions:**

- In a large bowl, combine cooked rice noodles, pan-fried tofu cubes, julienned cucumber, julienned carrots, thinly sliced red bell pepper, and chopped green onions.
- Drizzle with sesame oil and tamari.
- Sprinkle with sesame seeds.
- Toss gently to combine.
- Serve at room temperature.

**Serving Methods:**

1. Add a handful of mung bean sprouts for extra crunch.
2. Top with a squeeze of lime juice for a zesty kick.

# Low FODMAP Egg Salad Lettuce Wraps

**Ingredients:**

- Hard-boiled eggs, chopped
- Green leaf lettuce leaves
- Dijon mustard
- Olive oil
- Chives, chopped
- Salt and pepper to taste

**Preparation Time:** 10 minutes

***Serving Time:*** Immediate

***Nutritional Info:*** (per serving)

- Calories: 150
- Protein: 8g
- Healthy Fats: 11g

***Instructions:***

- In a bowl, combine chopped hard-boiled eggs, Dijon mustard, olive oil, chopped chives, salt, and pepper.
- Spoon the egg salad onto individual green leaf lettuce leaves.
- Serve immediately.

***Serving Methods:***

1. Add a slice of lactose-free cheese for added flavor.
2. Wrap in gluten-free tortillas for a portable lunch option.

## Low FODMAP Thai-Inspired Beef Salad

***Ingredients:***

- Beef sirloin, grilled and sliced
- Mixed salad greens
- Cucumber, thinly sliced
- Radishes, sliced
- Mint leaves

- Lime dressing (lime juice, fish sauce, and a touch of maple syrup)

**Preparation Time:** 15 minutes

**Cooking Time:** 10 minutes (for grilling beef)

**Serving Time:** Immediate

**Nutritional Info:** (per serving)

- Calories: 220
- Protein: 15g
- Healthy Fats: 10g

**Instructions:**

- Grill beef sirloin until cooked to your liking, then slice.
- In a bowl, combine mixed salad greens, thinly sliced cucumber, sliced radishes, and mint leaves.
- Drizzle with lime dressing.
- Toss gently to combine.
- Top with grilled beef slices.
- Serve at room temperature.

**Serving Methods:**

1. Sprinkle with crushed peanuts for added texture.
2. Garnish with cilantro for a burst of freshness.

# CHAPTER TEN

# MEAT AND POULTRY RECIPES

## Grilled Lemon Herb Chicken

*Ingredients:*

- Chicken breasts
- Lemon juice
- Olive oil
- Garlic-infused oil
- Fresh herbs (rosemary, thyme)
- Salt and pepper

*Preparation Time:* 10 minutes

*Cooking Time:* 15 minutes

*Serving Time:* Immediate

*Nutritional Info:* (per serving)

- Calories: 200
- Protein: 25g
- Healthy Fats: 10g

*Instructions:*

- Marinate chicken breasts in a mixture of lemon juice, olive oil, garlic-infused oil, fresh herbs, salt, and pepper.
- Grill until cooked through.
- Serve hot.

**Serving Methods:**

1. Slice and serve over a bed of quinoa.

2. Top with a dollop of lactose-free tzatziki for a refreshing twist.

# Low FODMAP Turkey and Zucchini Skewers

**Ingredients:**

- Ground turkey
- Zucchini, sliced
- Paprika
- Cumin
- Olive oil
- Salt and pepper

**Preparation Time:** 15 minutes

**Cooking Time:** 10 minutes

**Serving Time:** Immediate

**Nutritional Info:** (per serving)

- Calories: 180
- Protein: 20g
- Healthy Fats: 8g

**Instructions:**

- Mix ground turkey with paprika, cumin, olive oil, salt, and pepper.

- Thread turkey mixture and zucchini slices onto skewers.
- Grill until turkey is cooked through.
- Serve hot.

*Serving Methods:*

1. Serve over a bed of rice noodles.
2. Drizzle with a squeeze of lime for added freshness.

## Low FODMAP Herb-Crusted Pork Tenderloin

*Ingredients:*

- Pork tenderloin
- Dijon mustard
- Fresh herbs (parsley, thyme)
- Garlic-infused oil
- Salt and pepper

*Preparation Time:* 15 minutes

*Cooking Time:* 25 minutes

*Serving Time:* Immediate

*Nutritional Info:* (per serving)

- Calories: 220
- Protein: 30g
- Healthy Fats: 10g

*Instructions:*

- Coat pork tenderloin with Dijon mustard, fresh herbs, garlic-infused oil, salt, and pepper.
- Roast until the internal temperature reaches 145°F (63°C).
- Rest before slicing.
- Serve warm.

*Serving Methods:*

1. Pair with a side of roasted vegetables.
2. Drizzle with a balsamic reduction for added flavor.

## Low FODMAP Spaghetti Bolognese

*Ingredients:*

- Ground beef
- Gluten-free spaghetti
- Canned tomatoes
- Carrots, grated
- Olive oil
- Italian herbs
- Salt and pepper

*Preparation Time:* 20 minutes

*Cooking Time:* 30 minutes

*Serving Time:* Immediate

*Nutritional Info:* (per serving)

- Calories: 250
- Protein: 20g
- Fiber: 3g

*Instructions:*

- Brown ground beef in olive oil.
- Add grated carrots, canned tomatoes, Italian herbs, salt, and pepper.
- Simmer until flavors meld.
- Serve over cooked gluten-free spaghetti.

*Serving Methods:*

1. Top with grated Parmesan cheese.
2. Serve with a side of mixed green salad.

## Low FODMAP Grilled Salmon with Lemon-Dill Sauce

*Ingredients:*

- Salmon fillets
- Lemon zest
- Fresh dill, chopped
- Olive oil
- Salt and pepper

*Preparation Time:* 10 minutes

*Cooking Time:* 15 minutes

*Serving Time:* Immediate

***Nutritional Info:*** (per serving)

- Calories: 230
- Protein: 25g
- Healthy Fats: 12g

***Instructions:***

- Rub salmon fillets with lemon zest, fresh dill, olive oil, salt, and pepper.
- Grill until salmon flakes easily.
- Serve hot with lemon-dill sauce.

***Serving Methods:***

1. Serve over a bed of quinoa.
2. Pair with steamed asparagus for a complete meal.

# Low FODMAP Chicken and Vegetable Stir-Fry

***Ingredients:***

- Chicken breast, sliced
- Bell peppers, sliced
- Carrots, julienned
- Zucchini, sliced
- Tamari (gluten-free soy sauce)
- Sesame oil
- Ginger, grated

***Preparation Time:*** 15 minutes

***Cooking Time:*** 10 minutes

***Serving Time:*** Immediate

***Nutritional Info:*** (per serving)

- Calories: 180
- Protein: 20g
- Healthy Fats: 8g

***Instructions:***

- Stir-fry sliced chicken in sesame oil until cooked.
- Add sliced bell peppers, julienned carrots, and sliced zucchini.
- Stir in tamari and grated ginger.
- Cook until vegetables are tender.
- Serve hot.

***Serving Methods:***

1. Pair with jasmine rice.
2. Garnish with chopped green onions for extra flavor.

## Low FODMAP Rosemary and Lemon Roast Chicken

***Ingredients:***

- Whole chicken
- Rosemary, chopped
- Lemon juice
- Olive oil

- Garlic-infused oil
- Salt and pepper

*Preparation Time:* 15 minutes

*Cooking Time:* 1 hour and 30 minutes

*Serving Time:* Immediate

*Nutritional Info:* (per serving)

- Calories: 280
- Protein: 30g
- Healthy Fats: 15g

*Instructions:*

- Rub whole chicken with chopped rosemary, lemon juice, olive oil, garlic-infused oil, salt, and pepper.
- Roast until the internal temperature reaches 165°F (74°C).
- Let it rest before carving.
- Serve warm.

*Serving Methods:*

1. Pair with mashed potatoes.
2. Serve with a side of steamed green beans.

# Low FODMAP Maple Glazed Pork Chops

*Ingredients:*

- Pork chops
- Maple syrup

- Dijon mustard
- Olive oil
- Rosemary, chopped
- Salt and pepper

**Preparation Time:** 10 minutes

**Cooking Time:** 20 minutes

**Serving Time:** Immediate

**Nutritional Info:** (per serving)
- Calories: 250
- Protein: 25g
- Healthy Fats: 12g

**Instructions:**
- Mix maple syrup, Dijon mustard, olive oil, chopped rosemary, salt, and pepper.
- Brush the mixture over pork chops.
- Grill or pan-sear until fully cooked.
- Serve hot.

**Serving Methods:**
1. Pair with a side of roasted sweet potatoes.
2. Drizzle with additional maple glaze for extra sweetness.

# Low FODMAP Lemon Garlic Shrimp Skewers

**Ingredients:**

- Shrimp, peeled and deveined
- Lemon zest
- Garlic-infused oil
- Paprika
- Salt and pepper

**Preparation Time:** 15 minutes

**Cooking Time:** 8 minutes

**Serving Time:** Immediate

**Nutritional Info:** (per serving)

- Calories: 160
- Protein: 20g
- Healthy Fats: 8g

**Instructions:**

- Marinate shrimp in lemon zest, garlic-infused oil, paprika, salt, and pepper.
- Thread onto skewers and grill until opaque.
- Serve hot.

**Serving Methods:**

1. Serve over a bed of quinoa.
2. Pair with a side of grilled vegetables.

## Low FODMAP Teriyaki Chicken Skewers

**Ingredients:**

- Chicken thighs, cubed

- Pineapple chunks
- Teriyaki sauce (low FODMAP)
- Sesame seeds
- Green onions, chopped (green parts only)

*Preparation Time:* 15 minutes

*Cooking Time:* 12 minutes

*Serving Time:* Immediate

*Nutritional Info:* (per serving)

- Calories: 230
- Protein: 25g
- Healthy Fats: 10g

*Instructions:*

- Marinate chicken cubes in low FODMAP teriyaki sauce.
- Thread chicken and pineapple onto skewers.
- Grill until chicken is cooked.
- Sprinkle with sesame seeds and green onions.
- Serve hot.

*Serving Methods:*

1. Pair with jasmine rice.
2. Serve with a side of pickled ginger for added flavor.

# Low FODMAP Mustard and Herb Grilled Lamb Chops

### Ingredients:

- Lamb chops
- Dijon mustard
- Fresh herbs (rosemary, thyme)
- Olive oil
- Salt and pepper

**Preparation Time:** 15 minutes

**Cooking Time:** 12 minutes

**Serving Time:** Immediate

**Nutritional Info:** (per serving)

- Calories: 260
- Protein: 30g
- Healthy Fats: 15g

### Instructions:

- Mix Dijon mustard, fresh herbs, olive oil, salt, and pepper.
- Coat lamb chops with the mixture.
- Grill until lamb is cooked to your liking.
- Serve hot.

### Serving Methods:

1. Pair with a side of roasted Brussels sprouts.
2. Drizzle with balsamic reduction for added richness.

# Low FODMAP Lemon Herb Baked Cod

*Ingredients:*

- Cod fillets
- Lemon juice
- Fresh parsley, chopped
- Olive oil
- Garlic-infused oil
- Salt and pepper

*Preparation Time:* 10 minutes

*Baking Time:* 15 minutes

*Serving Time:* Immediate

*Nutritional Info:* (per serving)

- Calories: 180
- Protein: 22g
- Healthy Fats: 8g

*Instructions:*

- Place cod fillets in a baking dish.
- Drizzle with lemon juice, fresh parsley, olive oil, garlic-infused oil, salt, and pepper.
- Bake until cod is flaky.
- Serve warm.

*Serving Methods:*

1. Pair with a side of quinoa.

2. Top with a squeeze of fresh lemon for extra zing.

## Low FODMAP Cumin-Spiced Grilled Chicken Thighs

*Ingredients:*

- Chicken thighs, boneless and skinless
- Cumin
- Paprika
- Olive oil
- Lemon juice
- Salt and pepper

*Preparation Time:* 15 minutes

*Cooking Time:* 20 minutes

*Serving Time:* Immediate

*Nutritional Info:* (per serving)

- Calories: 210
- Protein: 25g
- Healthy Fats: 12g

*Instructions:*

- Rub chicken thighs with cumin, paprika, olive oil, lemon juice, salt, and pepper.
- Grill until fully cooked.
- Serve hot.

*Serving Methods:*

1. Pair with a side of sautéed spinach.
2. Drizzle with a tahini dressing for added richness.

# Low FODMAP Rosemary and Garlic Beef Skewers

*Ingredients:*

- Beef sirloin, cubed
- Rosemary, chopped
- Garlic-infused oil
- Balsamic vinegar
- Salt and pepper

*Preparation Time:* 15 minutes

*Cooking Time:* 10 minutes

*Serving Time:* Immediate

*Nutritional Info:* (per serving

- Calories: 240
- Protein: 28g
- Healthy Fats: 14g

*Instructions:*

- Marinate beef cubes in chopped rosemary, garlic-infused oil, balsamic vinegar, salt, and pepper.
- Thread onto skewers and grill until desired doneness.
- Serve hot.

1. Pair with a side of roasted sweet potatoes.
2. Drizzle with extra balsamic reduction for enhanced flavor.

## Low FODMAP Mediterranean Chicken Thighs

*Ingredients:*

- Chicken thighs, bone-in and skin-on
- Cherry tomatoes, halved
- Kalamata olives, pitted
- Fresh oregano, chopped
- Olive oil
- Lemon juice
- Salt and pepper

*Preparation Time:* 15 minutes

*Cooking Time:* 30 minutes

*Serving Time:* Immediate

*Nutritional Info:* (per serving)

- Calories: 250
- Protein: 26g
- Healthy Fats: 15g

*Instructions:*

- Arrange chicken thighs in a baking dish.

- Add halved cherry tomatoes and pitted Kalamata olives.
- Drizzle with olive oil, lemon juice, chopped oregano, salt, and pepper.
- Bake until chicken is cooked through.
- Serve warm.

**Serving Methods:**

1. Serve over a bed of quinoa.
2. Top with crumbled feta for added richness.

# CHAPTER ELEVEN

## Lemon Garlic Grilled Shrimp

*Ingredients:*

- Shrimp, peeled and deveined
- Lemon juice
- Garlic-infused oil
- Fresh parsley, chopped
- Salt and pepper

*Preparation Time:* 10 minutes

*Cooking Time:* 5 minutes

*Serving Time:* Immediate

*Nutritional Info:* (per serving)

- Calories: 150
- Protein: 20g
- Healthy Fats: 8g

*Instructions:*

- Marinate shrimp in lemon juice, garlic-infused oil, chopped parsley, salt, and pepper.
- Grill until shrimp are opaque.
- Serve hot.

*Serving Methods:*

1. Serve over a bed of quinoa.

2. Pair with a side of roasted vegetables.

# Low FODMAP Baked Cod with Herb Crust

**Ingredients:**

- Cod fillets
- Dijon mustard
- Fresh herbs (dill, chives)
- Olive oil
- Lemon zest
- Salt and pepper

**Preparation Time:** 15 minutes

**Baking Time:** 15 minutes

**Serving Time:** Immediate

**Nutritional Info:** (per serving)

- Calories: 180
- Protein: 22g
- Healthy Fats: 9g

**Instructions:**

- Mix Dijon mustard, fresh herbs, olive oil, lemon zest, salt, and pepper.
- Coat cod fillets with the mixture.
- Bake until cod is flaky.
- Serve warm.

**Serving Methods:**

1. Pair with a side of sautéed spinach.
2. Drizzle with a lemon-butter sauce for added richness.

## Low FODMAP Shrimp and Zucchini Noodles

*Ingredients:*
- Shrimp, peeled and deveined
- Zucchini, spiralized
- Cherry tomatoes, halved
- Olive oil
- Garlic-infused oil
- Basil, chopped
- Red pepper flakes (optional)

*Preparation Time:* 15 minutes

*Cooking Time:* 10 minutes

*Serving Time:* Immediate

*Nutritional Info:* (per serving)
- Calories: 160
- Protein: 18g
- Healthy Fats: 8g

*Instructions:*
- Sauté shrimp in olive oil and garlic-infused oil until cooked.
- Add zucchini noodles and cherry tomatoes.

- Cook until zucchini noodles are tender.
- Sprinkle with chopped basil and red pepper flakes.
- Serve hot.

**Serving Methods:**

1. Top with grated Parmesan cheese.
2. Serve over a bed of rice for a heartier meal.

# Low FODMAP Grilled Salmon with Dill Sauce

**Ingredients:**

- Salmon fillets
- Fresh dill, chopped
- Lactose-free yogurt
- Lemon juice
- Olive oil
- Salt and pepper

**Preparation Time:** 10 minutes

**Cooking Time:** 15 minutes

**Serving Time:** Immediate

**Nutritional Info:** (per serving)

- Calories: 220
- Protein: 25g
- Healthy Fats: 12g

**Instructions:**

- Mix chopped dill, lactose-free yogurt, lemon juice, olive oil, salt, and pepper to make the sauce.
- Grill salmon fillets until cooked through.
- Top with dill sauce.
- Serve hot.

*Serving Methods:*
1. Pair with a side of quinoa.
2. Serve over a bed of mixed greens for a light meal.

## Low FODMAP Tuna and Avocado Salad

*Ingredients:*
- Canned tuna, drained
- Avocado, diced
- Cucumber, diced
- Green olives, sliced
- Olive oil
- Lemon juice
- Chives, chopped
- Salt and pepper

*Preparation Time:* 10 minutes

*Serving Time:* Immediate

*Nutritional Info:* (per serving)
- Calories: 200
- Protein: 20g

- Healthy Fats: 12g

**Instructions:**

- In a bowl, combine drained tuna, diced avocado, diced cucumber, and sliced green olives.
- Drizzle with olive oil and lemon juice.
- Add chopped chives, salt, and pepper.
- Toss gently to combine.
- Serve chilled.

**Serving Methods:**

1. Scoop onto gluten-free crackers for a snack.
2. Wrap in lettuce leaves for a low-carb option.

# Low FODMAP Seared Scallops with Lemon Butter Sauce

**Ingredients:**

- Scallops
- Lemon zest
- Butter
- Chives, chopped
- Olive oil
- Salt and pepper

**Preparation Time:** 10 minutes

**Cooking Time:** 5 minutes

**Serving Time:** Immediate

*Nutritional Info:* (per serving)

- Calories: 180
- Protein: 20g
- Healthy Fats: 10g

*Instructions:*

- Pat scallops dry and season with salt and pepper.
- Sear in olive oil until golden brown on each side.
- In a separate pan, melt butter, add lemon zest, and chopped chives.
- Pour lemon butter sauce over seared scallops.
- Serve hot.

*Serving Methods:*

1. Pair with a side of sautéed spinach.
2. Serve over a bed of risotto for a luxurious meal.

## Low FODMAP Lemon Herb Grilled Swordfish

*Ingredients:*

- Swordfish steaks
- Lemon juice
- Fresh herbs (rosemary, thyme)
- Garlic-infused oil
- Salt and pepper

*Preparation Time:* 15 minutes

*Cooking Time:* 10 minutes

***Serving Time:*** Immediate

***Nutritional Info:*** (per serving)

- Calories: 250
- Protein: 30g
- Healthy Fats: 12g

***Instructions:***

- Marinate swordfish steaks in lemon juice, fresh herbs, garlic-infused oil, salt, and pepper.
- Grill until swordfish is cooked through.
- Serve hot.

***Serving Methods:***

1. Pair with a side of quinoa salad.
2. Top with a mango salsa for a tropical twist.

# Low FODMAP Baked Halibut with Tomato-Caper Relish

***Ingredients:***

- Halibut fillets
- Tomatoes, diced
- Capers, chopped
- Olive oil
- Lemon juice
- Fresh basil, chopped
- Salt and pepper

***Preparation Time:*** 15 minutes

***Baking Time:*** 20 minutes

***Serving Time:*** Immediate

***Nutritional Info:*** (per serving)

- Calories: 190
- Protein: 22g
- Healthy Fats: 10g

***Instructions:***

- Place halibut fillets in a baking dish.
- In a bowl, combine diced tomatoes, chopped capers, olive oil, lemon juice, fresh basil, salt, and pepper to make the relish.
- Spoon the relish over the halibut.
- Bake until fish is flaky.
- Serve warm.

***Serving Methods:***

1. Pair with a side of quinoa.
2. Serve over a bed of steamed asparagus.

# Low FODMAP Cajun Shrimp Skewers

***Ingredients:***

- Shrimp, peeled and deveined
- Cajun seasoning (low FODMAP)
- Olive oil

- Lemon wedges
- Fresh parsley, chopped
- Salt and pepper

**Preparation Time:** 10 minutes

**Cooking Time:** 5 minutes

**Serving Time:** Immediate

**Nutritional Info:** (per serving)

- Calories: 160
- Protein: 18g
- Healthy Fats: 9g

**Instructions:**

- Toss shrimp in olive oil and low FODMAP Cajun seasoning.
- Thread onto skewers and grill until shrimp are opaque.
- Sprinkle with chopped parsley, salt, and pepper.
- Serve hot with lemon wedges.

**Serving Methods:**

- Serve over a bed of rice.
- Top with a dollop of lactose-free sour cream.

# Low FODMAP Garlic and Herb Baked Salmon

**Ingredients:**

- Salmon fillets

- Garlic-infused oil
- Fresh herbs (parsley, dill)
- Lemon slices
- Salt and pepper

**Preparation Time:** 10 minutes

**Baking Time:** 15 minutes

**Serving Time:** Immediate

**Nutritional Info:** (per serving)

- Calories: 210
- Protein: 24g
- Healthy Fats: 12g

**Instructions:**

- Preheat the oven and line a baking dish with lemon slices.
- Place salmon fillets on the lemon slices.
- Drizzle with garlic-infused oil, sprinkle with fresh herbs, salt, and pepper.
- Bake until salmon is flaky.
- Serve warm.

**Serving Methods:**

1. Pair with a side of quinoa and roasted vegetables.
2. Top with a squeeze of fresh lemon for extra brightness.

# Low FODMAP Lemon Garlic Butter Shrimp Pasta

*Ingredients:*

- Shrimp, peeled and deveined
- Gluten-free pasta
- Garlic-infused oil
- Butter
- Lemon juice
- Fresh parsley, chopped
- Red pepper flakes (optional)

*Preparation Time:* 15 minutes

*Cooking Time:* 15 minutes

*Serving Time:* Immediate

*Nutritional Info:* (per serving)

- Calories: 280
- Protein: 22g
- Healthy Fats: 14g

*Instructions:*

- Cook gluten-free pasta according to package instructions.
- Sauté shrimp in garlic-infused oil and butter until cooked.
- Toss cooked pasta with shrimp, lemon juice, chopped parsley, and red pepper flakes.

- Serve warm.

***Serving Methods:***

1. Top with grated Parmesan cheese.
2. Garnish with extra chopped parsley.

# Low FODMAP Coconut Lime Grilled Shrimp

***Ingredients:***

- Shrimp, peeled and deveined
- Coconut milk (unsweetened)
- Lime zest
- Cilantro, chopped
- Olive oil
- Salt and pepper

***Preparation Time:*** 15 minutes

***Cooking Time:*** 5 minutes

***Serving Time:*** Immediate

***Nutritional Info:*** (per serving)

- Calories: 170
- Protein: 20g
- Healthy Fats: 8g

***Instructions:***

- Marinate shrimp in coconut milk, lime zest, chopped cilantro, olive oil, salt, and pepper.
- Grill until shrimp are opaque.

- Serve hot.

**Serving Methods:**

1. Pair with a side of coconut rice.

2. Top with a mango salsa for a tropical twist.

# Low FODMAP Tuscan Grilled Swordfish

**Ingredients:**

- Swordfish steaks
- Cherry tomatoes, halved
- Kalamata olives, pitted and sliced
- Fresh basil, chopped
- Olive oil
- Lemon juice
- Salt and pepper

**Preparation Time:** 15 minutes

**Cooking Time:** 10 minutes

**Serving Time:** Immediate

**Nutritional Info:** (per serving)

- Calories: 240
- Protein: 28g
- Healthy Fats: 12g

**Instructions:**

- Marinate swordfish steaks in olive oil, lemon juice, salt, and pepper.

- Grill until swordfish is cooked through.
- In a bowl, combine halved cherry tomatoes, sliced Kalamata olives, and chopped fresh basil.
- Spoon the mixture over the grilled swordfish.
- Serve hot.

*Serving Methods:*
1. Serve over a bed of quinoa.
2. Drizzle with balsamic glaze for added richness.

## Low FODMAP Lemon Herb Baked Shrimp

*Ingredients:*
- Shrimp, peeled and deveined
- Lemon juice
- Fresh herbs (thyme, rosemary)
- Olive oil
- Garlic-infused oil
- Salt and pepper

*Preparation Time:* 10 minutes
*Baking Time:* 15 minutes
*Serving Time:* Immediate
*Nutritional Info:* (per serving)
- Calories: 160
- Protein: 18g
- Healthy Fats: 8g

*Instructions:*

- Preheat the oven and line a baking dish with parchment paper.
- Place shrimp in the dish.
- Drizzle with lemon juice, fresh herbs, olive oil, garlic-infused oil, salt, and pepper.
- Bake until shrimp are opaque.
- Serve warm.

*Serving Methods:*

1. Pair with a side of quinoa.
2. Serve over a bed of sautéed spinach.

# Low FODMAP Miso Glazed Salmon

*Ingredients:*

- Salmon fillets
- Miso paste (low FODMAP)
- Maple syrup
- Rice vinegar
- Sesame oil
- Green onions, chopped (green parts only)

*Preparation Time:* 15 minutes

*Baking Time:* 15 minutes

*Serving Time:* Immediate

*Nutritional Info:* (per serving)

- Calories: 220
- Protein: 25g
- Healthy Fats: 12g

*Instructions:*

- Preheat the oven and line a baking sheet with parchment paper.
- In a bowl, mix miso paste, maple syrup, rice vinegar, and sesame oil to create the glaze.
- Brush the glaze over salmon fillets.
- Bake until salmon is cooked through.
- Garnish with chopped green onions.
- Serve warm.

*Serving Methods:*

1. Pair with a side of jasmine rice.
2. Top with sesame seeds for added texture.

# CHAPTER TWELVE

## MEAL PLAN

**Day 1:**

*Breakfast:* Lemon Garlic Grilled Shrimp

*Lunch:* Low FODMAP Tuna and Avocado Salad

*Dinner:* Low FODMAP Coconut Lime Grilled Shrimp

*Snack:* Fresh strawberries

*Dessert:* Low FODMAP Lemon Herb Baked Shrimp

## Day 2:

*Breakfast:* Low FODMAP Baked Cod with Herb Crust

*Lunch:* Low FODMAP Seared Scallops with Lemon Butter Sauce

*Dinner:* Low FODMAP Garlic and Herb Baked Salmon

*Snack:* Carrot sticks with hummus

*Dessert:* Kiwi slices

## Day 3:

*Breakfast:* Low FODMAP Shrimp and Zucchini Noodles

*Lunch:* Low FODMAP Tuscan Grilled Swordfish

*Dinner:* Low FODMAP Lemon Herb Grilled Swordfish

*Snack:* Lactose-free yogurt with blueberries

*Dessert:* Low FODMAP Miso Glazed Salmon

## Day 4:

*Breakfast:* Low FODMAP Lemon Herb Baked Cod

*Lunch:* Low FODMAP Baked Halibut with Tomato-Caper Relish

*Dinner:* Low FODMAP Cajun Shrimp Skewers

*Snack:* Almonds

*Dessert:* Dark chocolate squares

## Day 5:

*Breakfast:* Low FODMAP Tuna and Avocado Salad

*Lunch:* Low FODMAP Rosemary and Garlic Beef Skewers

*Dinner:* Low FODMAP Teriyaki Chicken Skewers

*Snack:* Grapes

*Dessert:* Low FODMAP Thai-Inspired Beef Salad

## Day 6:

*Breakfast:* Low FODMAP Lemon Herb Grilled Swordfish

*Lunch:* Low FODMAP Cumin-Spiced Grilled Chicken Thighs

*Dinner:* Low FODMAP Baked Halibut with Tomato-Caper Relish

*Snack:* Cucumber slices with lactose-free cheese

*Dessert:* Pineapple slices

## Day 7:

*Breakfast:* Low FODMAP Baked Cod with Herb Crust
*Lunch:* Low FODMAP Coconut Lime Grilled Shrimp
*Dinner:* Low FODMAP Mustard and Herb Grilled Lamb Chops
*Snack:* Mixed nuts
*Dessert:* Mixed berries

## Day 8:

*Breakfast:* Low FODMAP Seared Scallops with Lemon Butter Sauce
*Lunch:* Low FODMAP Teriyaki Chicken Skewers
*Dinner:* Low FODMAP Lemon Herb Baked Shrimp
*Snack:* Rice cakes with almond butter
*Dessert:* Mango slices

## Day 9:

*Breakfast:* Low FODMAP Grilled Salmon with Dill Sauce
*Lunch:* Low FODMAP Baked Halibut with Tomato-Caper Relish
*Dinner:* Low FODMAP Lemon Garlic Butter Shrimp Pasta

Snack: Cherry tomatoes with balsamic glaze

*Dessert:* Low FODMAP Rosemary and Garlic Beef Skewers

## Day 10:

*Breakfast:* Low FODMAP Miso Glazed Salmon

*Lunch:* Low FODMAP Shrimp and Zucchini Noodles

*Dinner:* Low FODMAP Lemon Herb Baked Cod

Snack: Sliced bell peppers with guacamole

*Dessert:* Kiwi slices

## Day 11:

*Breakfast:* Low FODMAP Baked Halibut with Tomato-Caper Relish

*Lunch:* Low FODMAP Grilled Salmon with Dill Sauce

*Dinner:* Low FODMAP Garlic and Herb Baked Salmon

*Snack:* Lactose-free yogurt with raspberries

*Dessert:* Dark chocolate squares

## Day 12:

*Breakfast:* Low FODMAP Shrimp and Zucchini Noodles

*Lunch:* Low FODMAP Rosemary and Garlic Beef Skewers

*Dinner:* Low FODMAP Tuscan Grilled Swordfish

Snack: Almonds

*Dessert:* Fresh strawberries

*Day 13:*

*Breakfast:* Low FODMAP Mustard and Herb Grilled Lamb Chops

*Lunch:* Low FODMAP Tuna and Avocado Salad

*Dinner:* Low FODMAP Coconut Lime Grilled Shrimp

*Snack:* Carrot sticks with hummus

*Dessert:* Pineapple slices

## Day 14:

*Breakfast:* Low FODMAP Lemon Herb Baked Cod

*Lunch:* Low FODMAP Teriyaki Chicken Skewers

*Dinner:* Low FODMAP Baked Halibut with Tomato-Caper Relish

*Snack:* Mixed nuts

*Dessert:* Mixed berries

## Day 15:

*Breakfast:* Low FODMAP Lemon Herb Baked Shrimp

*Lunch:* Low FODMAP Shrimp and Zucchini Noodles

*Dinner:* Low FODMAP Lemon Herb Grilled Swordfish

*Snack:* Rice cakes with almond butter

*Dessert:* Mango slices

# Day 16:

*Breakfast:* Low FODMAP Grilled Salmon with Dill Sauce

*Lunch:* Low FODMAP Cajun Shrimp Skewers

*Dinner:* Low FODMAP Lemon Garlic Butter Shrimp Pasta

*Snack:* Cherry tomatoes with balsamic glaze

*Dessert:* Low FODMAP Rosemary and Garlic Beef Skewers

# Day 17:

*Breakfast:* Low FODMAP Baked Cod with Herb Crust

*Lunch:* Low FODMAP Tuna and Avocado Salad

*Dinner:* Low FODMAP Garlic and Herb Baked Salmon

*Snack:* Sliced bell peppers with guacamole

*Dessert:* Dark chocolate squares

# Day 18:

*Breakfast:* Low FODMAP Mustard and Herb Grilled Lamb Chops

*Lunch:* Low FODMAP Seared Scallops with Lemon Butter Sauce

*Dinner:* Low FODMAP Coconut Lime Grilled Shrimp

Snack: Almonds
*Dessert:* Fresh strawberries

## Day 19:

*Breakfast:* Low FODMAP Miso Glazed Salmon
*Lunch:* Low FODMAP Rosemary and Garlic Beef Skewers
*Dinner:* Low FODMAP Tuscan Grilled Swordfish
*Snack:* Lactose-free yogurt with raspberries
*Dessert:* Kiwi slices

## Day 20:

*Breakfast:* Low FODMAP Lemon Herb Baked Cod
*Lunch:* Low FODMAP Teriyaki Chicken Skewers
*Dinner:* Low FODMAP Baked Halibut with Tomato-Caper Relish
*Snack:* Carrot sticks with hummus
*Dessert:* Pineapple slices

## Day 21:

*Breakfast:* Low FODMAP Shrimp and Zucchini Noodles
*Lunch:* Low FODMAP Grilled Salmon with Dill Sauce
*Dinner:* Low FODMAP Lemon Herb Baked Shrimp
*Snack:* Mixed nuts

*Dessert:* Mixed berries

## Day 22:

*Breakfast:* Low FODMAP Rosemary and Garlic Beef Skewers

*Lunch:* Low FODMAP Baked Halibut with Tomato-Caper Relish

*Dinner:* Low FODMAP Garlic and Herb Baked Salmon

*Snack:* Rice cakes with almond butter

*Dessert:* Mango slices

## Day 23:

*Breakfast:* Low FODMAP Mustard and Herb Grilled Lamb Chops

*Lunch:* Low FODMAP Seared Scallops with Lemon Butter Sauce

*Dinner:* Low FODMAP Coconut Lime Grilled Shrimp

*Snack:* Cherry tomatoes with balsamic glaze

*Dessert:* Dark chocolate squares

## Day 24:

*Breakfast:* Low FODMAP Shrimp and Zucchini Noodles

*Lunch:* Low FODMAP Rosemary and Garlic Beef Skewers

*Dinner:* Low FODMAP Tuscan Grilled Swordfish

Snack: Almonds

*Dessert:* Fresh strawberries

## Day 25:

*Breakfast:* Low FODMAP Baked Cod with Herb Crust

*Lunch:* Low FODMAP Tuna and Avocado Salad

*Dinner:* Low FODMAP Lemon Garlic Butter Shrimp Pasta

*Snack:* Sliced bell peppers with guacamole

*Dessert:* Low FODMAP Rosemary and Garlic Beef Skewers

## Day 26:

*Breakfast:* Low FODMAP Lemon Herb Baked Shrimp

*Lunch:* Low FODMAP Teriyaki Chicken Skewers

*Dinner:* Low FODMAP Baked Halibut with Tomato-Caper Relish

*Snack:* Lactose-free yogurt with raspberries

*Dessert:* Kiwi slices

## Day 27:

*Breakfast:* Low FODMAP Grilled Salmon with Dill Sauce

*Lunch:* Low FODMAP Cajun Shrimp Skewers

*Dinner:* Low FODMAP Lemon Herb Baked Cod

*Snack:* Mixed nuts

*Dessert:* Mixed berries

## Day 28:

*Breakfast:* Low FODMAP Shrimp and Zucchini Noodles

*Lunch:* Low FODMAP Mustard and Herb Grilled Lamb Chops

*Dinner:* Low FODMAP Coconut Lime Grilled Shrimp

*Snack:* Carrot sticks with hummus

*Dessert:* Pineapple slices

## Day 29:

*Breakfast:* Low FODMAP Lemon Herb Baked Cod

*Lunch:* Low FODMAP Teriyaki Chicken Skewers

*Dinner:* Low FODMAP Garlic and Herb Baked Salmon

*Snack:* Rice cakes with almond butter

*Dessert:* Dark chocolate squares

## Day 30:

*Breakfast:* Low FODMAP Tuna and Avocado Salad

*Lunch:* Low FODMAP Rosemary and Garlic Beef Skewers

*Dinner:* Low FODMAP Tuscan Grilled Swordfish

**Snack:** Mixed nuts

**Dessert:** Fresh strawberries

# CHAPTER THIRTEEN
## MONITORING PROGRESS AND REINTRODUCING FODMAPS

## Tracking Symptoms

*Tracking symptoms is an essential aspect of managing the Low FODMAP Diet. Keeping a detailed record can help identify patterns, trigger foods, and improvements over time. Here's a guide on how to track symptoms:*

**Tracking Sheet:**
*Date:*

- Record the date for each entry.

*Meal:*

- Specify the meal (breakfast, lunch, dinner, snack).

*Food Consumed:*

- List all foods consumed, including ingredients and portion sizes.

*Symptoms:*

- Create a list of common symptoms (bloating, gas, abdominal pain, etc.).

- Use a scale (1-10) to rate the severity of each symptom.

**FODMAP Content:**

- Indicate the FODMAP content of each food item (High, Moderate, Low).

**Time of Onset:**

- Note when symptoms started after eating (immediately, 1 hour, 2 hours, etc.).

**Medication/Supplements:**

- Include any medications or supplements taken.

**Other Factors:**

- Consider external factors (stress, sleep, physical activity) that may influence symptoms.

## Tips for Effective Tracking:

### Consistency is Key:

- Track consistently, ideally for the entire duration of the Low FODMAP Diet.

### Be Detailed:

- Provide specific details about foods and ingredients.
- Include cooking methods and recipes.

### Include Beverages:

- Record beverages, as they can also impact symptoms.

**Use a Journal or App:**

- Consider using a dedicated journal or a mobile app for convenient tracking.

**Note Non-FODMAP Factors:**

- Record factors like stress, sleep, and physical activity, as they can affect symptoms.

**Include Positive Changes:**

- Document any improvements or positive changes in symptoms.

**Consult with a Professional:**

- Share your tracking sheet with a healthcare professional or dietitian for personalized insights.

**Example Tracking Entry:**

*Date:* 2024-03-01

*Meal:* Breakfast

*Food Consumed:*

- Low FODMAP Baked Cod with Herb Crust
- Quinoa (1/2 cup)

- Spinach Salad with Olive Oil Dressing

- Lemon-infused Water

## Symptoms:

- Bloating: 3/10

- Gas: 2/10

- Abdominal Pain: 1/10

## FODMAP Content:

- Baked Cod: Low

- Quinoa: Low

- Spinach: Low

## Time of Onset:

- Symptoms started 2 hours after the meal.

## Medication/Supplements:

- None

## Other Factors:

- Stress: Low

- Sleep: 7 hours

- Physical Activity: Moderate

## Analysis:

- The entry suggests a relatively low symptom severity, indicating that the meal may be well-tolerated.

- Identifying low FODMAP foods and favorable external factors may contribute to symptom management.

- Over time, patterns and trends can be observed, guiding adjustments to the diet.

## Gradual Reintroduction Process

*The gradual reintroduction process is a crucial phase of the Low FODMAP Diet. It involves systematically reintroducing specific FODMAP groups to identify individual tolerance levels and expand the variety of foods in your diet.*

**Here's a guide on how to approach the reintroduction process:**

**1. Understand the Reintroduction Phases:**

*Phase 1: Reintroduction*

- Reintroduce one FODMAP group at a time in small amounts.

- Allow a few days between reintroductions to monitor symptoms.

*Phase 2: Evaluation*

- Assess symptoms and record any reactions.
- Note the specific FODMAPs causing symptoms.

***Phase 3: Personalization***

- Customize your diet based on individual tolerance levels.
- Expand food choices while minimizing symptom triggers.

## 2. Selecting Foods for Reintroduction:

- Choose foods that belong to one FODMAP group (e.g., Fructans, Galacto-oligosaccharides, sorbitol).
- Begin with foods you miss or those you suspect may be better tolerated.

## 3. Reintroduction Schedule:

***Day 1-3:***

- Reintroduce a small amount of the chosen FODMAP group in the morning.
- Monitor for symptoms over the next 24-48 hours.

***Days 4-6:***

- Resume a strict Low FODMAP Diet to establish a baseline.
- Note any lingering symptoms.

***Days 7-9:***

- Reintroduce a different FODMAP group.

- Monitor symptoms.

*Repeat:*

- Continue the process with other FODMAP groups.

## 4. Monitoring Symptoms:

*Physical Symptoms:*

- Bloating, gas, abdominal pain, diarrhea, constipation.
- Rate symptom severity on a scale (1-10).

*Other Factors:*

- Consider stress levels, sleep, and physical activity.
- External factors may influence symptoms.

## 5. Recording Results:

*Symptom Journal:*

- Maintain a detailed journal for each reintroduction.
- Include the specific food, portion size, and symptom severity.

*Consult with a Professional:*

- Share reintroduction results with a healthcare professional or dietitian.
- Seek guidance on interpretation and next steps.

## 6. Personalization:

*Identify Tolerated Foods:*

- Note which foods are well-tolerated without triggering symptoms.

- Incorporate these into your regular diet.

***Limit Trigger Foods:***

- Identify specific FODMAPs causing symptoms.
- Limit or avoid foods high in those FODMAPs.

## 7. Examples of Reintroduction Foods:

***Fructans (e.g., wheat, onions):***

- Reintroduce a small portion of wheat-based products or onions.

**Galacto-oligosaccharides (e.g., legumes):**

- Reintroduce a small amount of lentils or chickpeas.

***Fructose (e.g., honey, apples):***

- Reintroduce a small portion of honey or an apple.

***Polyols (e.g., stone fruits, sweeteners):***

- Reintroduce a small amount of a polyol-containing food like cherries or sorbitol.

## 8. Seek Professional Guidance:

***Consult with a Dietitian:***

- Work with a registered dietitian for personalized guidance.
- Discuss individual responses and potential modifications.

### 9. Long-Term Dietary Strategy:

*Balanced Diet:*

- Aim for a balanced diet that includes a variety of foods.

- Emphasize tolerated foods while minimizing trigger foods.

*Regular Reassessments:*

- Periodically reassess tolerance levels and adjust the diet accordingly

## Seeking Professional Guidance

### 1. Consult with a Registered Dietitian:

*Find a Specialized Dietitian:*

- Look for a dietitian with expertise in gastrointestinal health and the Low FODMAP Diet.

*Credentials:*

- Ensure the dietitian is a registered dietitian (RD) or a registered dietitian nutritionist (RDN).

*Experience:*

- Inquire about their experience working with individuals on the Low FODMAP Diet.

### 2. Schedule an Initial Consultation:

*Preparation:*

- Gather information about your dietary history, symptoms, and any previous attempts at managing digestive issues.

*Discuss Goals:*

- Clearly communicate your goals, whether it's symptom relief, weight management, or improving overall digestive health.

### 3. During the Consultation:

*Symptom Assessment:*

- Discuss your current symptoms, their severity, and how they impact your daily life.

*Dietary Analysis:*

- Share your typical dietary habits and any challenges you've faced.

*Education:*

- Ensure the dietitian provides comprehensive education on the Low FODMAP Diet, including food lists, cooking tips, and label reading.

*Reintroduction Guidance:*

- If applicable, discuss the reintroduction phase and create a personalized plan.

## 4. Follow-Up Sessions:

### *Regular Check-Ins:*

- Schedule follow-up sessions to monitor progress, discuss challenges, and make necessary adjustments.

### *Review Reintroduction Results:*

- Analyze the results of the reintroduction phase and modify the diet accordingly.

## 5. Ask Questions:

### *Clarify Doubts:*

- Don't hesitate to ask questions about specific foods, cooking methods, or any aspect of the diet that you find confusing.

### *Discuss Concerns:*

- Share any concerns or difficulties you're experiencing during the diet.

## 6. Collaboration with Healthcare Team:

### *Coordinate with Healthcare Professionals:*

- If you have other medical conditions or are under the care of a healthcare team, ensure that your dietitian collaborates with them.

### *Medication Management:*

- Discuss any medications or supplements you are taking, as these may interact with dietary changes.

## 7. Monitor Non-Dietary Factors:
### *Address Non-FODMAP Factors:*
- Discuss the impact of stress, sleep, and physical activity on symptoms.

### *Holistic Approach:*
- Work towards a holistic approach that considers both dietary and lifestyle factors.

## 8. Long-Term Strategies:
### *Transition to Maintenance:*
- Plan for the transition from the elimination phase to a more varied and sustainable diet.

### *Nutrient Adequacy:*
- Ensure that your diet remains nutritionally adequate over the long term.

## 9. Stay Open to Adjustments:
### *Flexibility:*
- Be open to making adjustments based on your evolving needs and responses to the diet.

### *Problem-Solving:*

- Work with your dietitian to problem-solve challenges and find practical solutions.

## 10. Personalized Support:

*Tailored Advice:*

- Seek personalized advice based on your unique health history, preferences, and lifestyle.

*Advocacy:*

- Your dietitian should empower you to become an advocate for your own digestive health.

# CONCLUSION

In conclusion, embarking on the Low FODMAP Diet for beginners involves a systematic and well-informed approach to managing digestive symptoms. Understanding the principles of the diet, the gradual reintroduction process, and seeking professional guidance are key elements in achieving success and long-term digestive health.

The journey begins with a solid comprehension of the Low FODMAP Diet, including its definition, common types of FODMAPs, and how these fermentable carbohydrates affect the digestive system. Armed with this knowledge, individuals can better appreciate the nuances of FODMAP content in various foods, make informed choices, and optimize their dietary habits.

The importance of mental and physical preparation should not be overlooked. Preparing both mentally and physically for the diet transition sets the stage for a smoother experience, enabling individuals to navigate challenges with resilience and dedication. This mental readiness, coupled with an understanding of how to read food labels effectively, empowers individuals to make choices aligned with their dietary needs.

Crucially, consulting with a healthcare professional, particularly a registered dietitian with expertise in the Low FODMAP Diet, is a pivotal step. Professional guidance ensures a personalized approach, with tailored advice, regular check-ins, and the expertise to navigate the intricacies of the diet. It also allows for the incorporation of a holistic view, considering non-dietary factors that may influence digestive health.

The reintroduction process marks a significant phase in the Low FODMAP Diet, as it provides the opportunity to identify individual tolerance levels and expand the variety of foods in the diet. Diligently tracking symptoms, recording results, and seeking professional interpretation are essential components of this phase. Through this systematic process, individuals can customize their diet, including tolerated foods and limiting trigger foods, fostering a sustainable and balanced approach to nutrition.

To further support the journey, a 30-day meal plan was provided, offering a diverse range of recipes for breakfast, lunch, dinner, snacks, and dessert. These recipes not only align with the Low FODMAP principles but also ensure nutritional adequacy and delicious variety, enhancing the overall dining experience for those on the diet.

In the long term, maintaining a balanced and varied diet, monitoring symptoms, and staying open to adjustments are key strategies for sustained success. Regular communication with healthcare professionals ensures ongoing support and guidance, contributing to the overall well-being of individuals following the Low FODMAP Diet.